W9-BID-366

LIPPINCOTT'S
Guide to Preventing Medication Errors

LIPPINCOTT'S
Guide to Preventing Medication Errors

AMY M. KARCH, RN, MS
Assistant Professor of Clinical Nursing
University of Rochester School of Nursing
New York

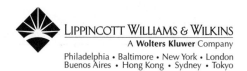

LIPPINCOTT WILLIAMS & WILKINS
A **Wolters Kluwer** Company

Philadelphia • Baltimore • New York • London
Buenos Aires • Hong Kong • Sydney • Tokyo

STAFF

Publisher
Judith A. Schilling McCann, RN, MSN

Editorial Director
H. Nancy Holmes

Clinical Director
Joan M. Robinson, RN, MSN

Senior Art Director
Arlene Putterman

Clinical Editors
Kate McGovern, RN, MSN, CCRN (project manager);
Melissa M. Devlin, PHARMD

Editors
Jennifer P. Kowalak (senior associate editor),
William Welsh (associate editor),
Naina D. Chohan, Kate Jackson

Copy Editors
Kimberly Bilotta,
Amy Furman, Dona Hightower,
Dorothy Terry, Pamela Wingrod

Cover Design
Tom Jackson

Digital Composition Services
Diane Paluba (manager),
Joyce Rossi Biletz (senior desktop assistant),
Donna S. Morris

Manufacturing
Patricia Dorshaw (senior manager),
Beth Janae Orr (book production coordinator)

Editorial Assistants
Danielle J. Barsky, Beverly Lane, Linda Ruhf

Librarian
Catherine M. Heslin

Indexer
Ellen S. Brennan

The clinical procedures described and recommended in this publication are based on research and consultation with medical and nursing authorities. To the best of our knowledge, these procedures reflect currently accepted clinical practice; nevertheless, they can't be considered absolute and universal recommendations. For individual application, treatment recommendations must be considered in light of the patient's clinical condition and, before administration of new or infrequently used drugs, in light of the latest package-insert information. The authors and the publisher disclaim responsibility for any adverse effects resulting directly or indirectly from the suggested procedures, from any undetected errors, or from the reader's misunderstanding of the text.

LGPME – D N O S A J J M A M F J
04   10 9 8 7 6 5 4 3 2

Library of Congress
Cataloging-in-Publication Data

Karch, Amy Morrison, 1949–
Lippincott's guide to preventing medication errors / Amy M. Karch.
   p. ; cm.
Includes index.
   1. Medication errors. 2. Nursing.
   [DNLM: 1. Medication Errors – prevention & control – Handbooks. QV 39 K18L 2003]
I. Title: Guide to preventing medication errors. II. Title.
RM146 .K37 2003
615'.1–dc21
ISBN 1-58255-185-5 (pbk. : alk. paper)   2002013937

Contents

Consultants

Melody C. Antoon, RN, MSN
Instructor-School of Nursing, Lamar University,
Beaumont, Tex.

Cheryl L. Brady, RN, MSN
Adjunct Faculty, Kent State University,
E. Liverpool, Ohio

Sandra H. Clark, RN, MSN
Assistant Professor, Armstrong Atlantic State University,
Savannah, Ga.

Marsha L. Conroy, RN, MSN, APN
Nursing Instructor, Cuyahoga Community College,
Cleveland

Margaret M. Gingrich, RN, MSN
Associate Professor, Harrisburg (Pa.) Area Community
College

Sandra Liming, RN, MN, PhC
Practical Nursing Program Coordinator/Instructor,
North Seattle (Wash.) Community College

Terri M. Perkins, RN, MN
Instructor, Associate Degree Nursing, Bellevue (Wash.)
Community College

Jo A. Voss, RN, PhD(C), CNS
Assistant Professor, South Dakota State University,
Rapid City

Preface

Whenever a medication is given to patient, there's always the possibility that an error could occur. The medication could be given to the wrong patient, it could be the wrong dose, it could be given by the wrong route, it could be given at the wrong time, or it could even be the wrong drug.

This isn't a new problem. The potential for error has existed since medications were first used to treat patients. Today, however, the possibility of error is greater than ever before because more drugs are available, more people are being treated with drugs, and more patients are taking more combinations of drugs. Add to this the current severe shortage of nurses and pharmacists in this country. Those who are working are frequently stressed, overworked, and fatigued. A situation like this increases the likelihood of an error. Patients are concerned about their personal safety. Health care providers are concerned about the health and welfare of the patients in their care. Hospitals and insurance companies are concerned about the ultimate financial cost of medication errors.

The antidote is the book you hold in your hands: *Lippincott's Guide to Preventing Medication Errors.* This handy guide spotlights hundreds of real-life medication errors to show how easily errors can occur — and how easily they can be avoided. Graphic icons marked "Prevent it" point the way, and checklists serve as quick reminders of steps to review before administering a drug. Appendices provide a quick reference to dialyzable drugs, adverse reactions that can be mistaken for age-related changes in a patient, and antidotes for poisoning, overdose, and vesicant extravasation.

Nursing has traditionally used the five "rights" of drug administration — the right patient, right drug, right dose, right route, and right time — as quick and comprehensive guides to avoid medication errors. *Lippincott's Guide to Preventing Medication Errors* is logically organized by these five rights and offers a comprehensive and clinically useful review of what should be considered with each right. Reviewing the five rights before administering each drug can catch the problems that are responsible for most medication errors in clinical settings, help to reinforce the procedure, and ensure safe care for each patient.

The bottom line is that educated, responsible, and vigilant people are the best tools for preventing medication errors. Teaching health care providers how to be vigilant, giving them a useful and comprehensive guide to preventing medication errors, and periodically reinforcing what they've learned are important steps.

Teaching the *patient* to approach each drug dose with the five "rights" in mind adds another check on the process. Teaching him to be his own advocate, to keep records, and to ask questions is equally essential. Because educating and supporting the patient is usually the nurse's job, this book's summary chapter offers guidelines and helpful hints for effective patient teaching.

Treating patients who have experienced a medication error can be costly not only in health care expenditures but in time. It can delay treatment of the original problem or cause adverse effects that are unpleasant, detrimental, or even fatal. Educated and vigilant nurses, prescribers, pharmacists, and patients are the key to conquering this serious problem. With everyone working together, using the five rights as a guide, medication errors can be controlled and reduced.

Amy M. Karch, RN, MS

Chapter

Issues in safe medication practice

A medication error is an incident in which a patient receives the wrong drug or receives the right drug but by the wrong route, at the wrong dose, or at the wrong time. Some of these errors can be life-threatening; however, in most cases they may cause some discomfort or prolong an illness, leading to additional therapy or a new set of adverse effects with which a patient needs to cope.

In recent years, the increasing rate of reported medication errors has become a headline issue. Among the factors believed to contribute to the increase of error reports are overworked health care providers, a severe shortage of nurses and pharmacists despite a steadily increasing number of patients, and the availability of a wide range of heavily promoted drugs. The ease of contacting various national reporting centers for adverse effects may also account for the growing numbers of reported errors. (See *Social factors in medication errors*, page 2.)

The health care system has several built-in checks and counterchecks to detect potential errors and to increase the safety of drug therapy. Physicians, pharmacists, patients, and nurses all share responsibility for preventing medication errors in the following ways:

Social factors in medication errors

Further complicating the medication situation is a patient's free access to a vast source of medical and pharmacologic information on the Internet — accurate as well as inaccurate. The media are overloaded with advertisements for prescription drugs, even offering money-saving coupons for using particular drugs.

The media also provide plenty of free medical and diagnostic advice, only some of which is based on scientific data. Alternative therapies, such as herbal aids and dietary supplements, are being widely promoted as the best and most natural way for people to take control of their health care. The fact that they may interact negatively with prescription drugs is rarely clear.

The availability of over-the-counter (OTC) drugs allows unsupervised use of many compounds that once were regulated by health care providers. Use of these drugs may mask signs and symptoms, which could result in incorrect diagnoses. Also, OTC drugs frequently interact with each other and with prescription drugs.

Further complicating the picture are the skyrocketing financial costs associated with health care and drug therapy. Health care providers must now contend with patients who demand specific treatments or specific drugs that they've read about or researched, who self-treat with a variety of OTC drugs and alternative therapies, and who insist that their health care costs be held in check. "Routine" drug therapy is no longer routine.

✦ The physician or other prescriber determines the prescribed medication and its route, dose, and timing.
✦ The pharmacist filling the prescription checks to make sure that the requested drug is labeled for the right patient, in the right dose, and by the

right route. The pharmacist may face obstacles to communication such as difficulty reading or comprehending the prescription. In many facilities, the pharmacist is also able to crosscheck other medications the patient may be receiving to make sure that interactions aren't a prohibiting factor.

✦ The patient, if he's alert and oriented, should be responsible for knowing the names, dosages, and timing of all his medications, asking about the purpose of each drug, and making sure that the drugs he receives are intended for him.

✦ During the discharge phase of hospitalization, the nurse, frequently the last check in the system, is generally responsible for administering prescribed drugs to the patient and is usually the person who instructs the patient in home management of potentially complicated drug regimens.

✦ The five "rights" rule

The underlying rationale for safe nursing drug administration has always been the five "rights" — the right patient, right drug, right dose, right route, and right time. When a nursing medication error occurs, it's because of a problem with one of these five issues. The monumental task of preventing medication errors can be accomplished in everyday clinical practice by applying the five rights to each and every drug preparation for patient administration. It doesn't take long to apply the rights, and with continued practice, the use of this proven safeguard against medication errors will become second nature.

The basic rule that all nurses can follow to help ensure the safety of drug therapy and to prevent medication errors is very simple: "When in doubt, check it out." Never assume that you can know all the drugs, all the drug effects, all the doses, all the routes, and all of the timing implications. Drug therapy practices change daily — indications, dosages, warnings, and routes. If something doesn't look familiar, if it seems not to fit, or if it seems odd, look it up, check with another nurse, your supervisor, or the pharmacist, and verify the information. Assure yourself that it's the right drug for the right patient at the right dose by the right route at the right time.

This book will look at the five rights for nursing drug administration and offer spot checks within each right to prevent medication errors.

✦ Drugs and drug therapy

The human body works as the result of a complicated series of chemical reactions and processes. Drugs, by definition, are chemicals that are introduced into the body to cause some sort of change. When drugs are administered, the body undergoes a series of reactions, which involves breakdown of the drug, use of the chemicals by the body's cells and, finally, elimination of the drug. When these reactions begin, they in turn affect the body's complex series of chemical reactions.

Understanding how drugs in the body cause changes and applying that knowledge in the clinical setting are important aspects of nursing practice. Patients often follow complicated drug regimens and receive potentially toxic drugs; many also manage their own care at home. The nurse is in a unique position to assist them with drug therapy because nursing responsibilities include:

- ✦ administering drugs
- ✦ assessing drug effects
- ✦ intervening to make the drug regimen more tolerable
- ✦ providing patient teaching about drugs and the drug regimen.

All of these responsibilities fall under the branch of science called pharmacotherapeutics, or clinical pharmacology. This is the study of drugs as they're used to treat, prevent, or diagnose disease. Clinical pharmacology addresses two key concerns: the drug's effects on the body and the body's response to the drug. Knowledge of a drug's intended action; how it's absorbed, eliminated, and dispensed; its potential adverse effects; and appropriate nursing considerations makes these responsibilities easier to perform, thus enhancing drug therapy.

Drug development

Chemicals that might prove useful as drugs can come from many natural sources, such as plants, animals, or inorganic compounds. They may also be developed from synthetic sources. To be used as a drug, a chemical must produce a demonstrated therapeutic value or efficacy without severe toxicity or damaging properties. In the United States, the Food and Drug Administration (FDA) controls the process authorizing which chemicals become marketable drugs. The FDA is part of the U.S. Department of Health and Human Services and is responsible for the development, regulation, and sale of drugs. FDA-regulated tests are designed to ensure that a drug approved for use in the United States is safe and reliable. Public safety is the main concern of the various FDA committees that examine each proposed drug. Consequently, for every 100,000 chemicals that are identified as potential drugs, only an estimated 5 are ultimately marketed as drugs.

A chemical must pass through a series of studies, or trials, before it can be offered for sale as a drug. These include preclinical trials and phase I, II, and III clinical trials. Preclinical trials involve testing potential drugs on laboratory animals to determine their potential

✦

Phases of clinical trials

PHASE I STUDIES

These studies use human volunteers to test drugs and are more tightly con-trolled than preclinical trials. Specially trained clinical investigators who per-form these studies scrutinize the drugs' effects in humans and also look for adverse effects and toxicity. At the end of phase I studies, many chemicals are dropped from the testing and development process because:

✦ they lack therapeutic effect in humans
✦ they cause unacceptable adverse effects
✦ they're highly teratogenic
✦ they're too toxic.

PHASE II STUDIES

Phase II studies allow investigators to use the drugs in patients who have the diseases that the drugs are meant to treat. Patients are told of the pos-sible benefits of the drugs and are invited to participate in the studies. Those who consent are fully informed of possible risks and are followed very closely to evaluate the drugs' effects. At the end of phase II studies, drugs may be removed from further investigation because:

✦ they're less effective than anticipated
✦ they're too toxic when used in patients
✦ they produce unacceptable adverse effects
✦ they have a low benefit-to-risk ratio
✦ they're no more effective than drugs already on the market, making the cost of continued research and production less attractive to the drug companies.

PHASE III STUDIES

These studies involve using the drugs in vast clinical markets. Prescribers are informed of all known reactions to the drugs and precautions required for their safe use. They follow patients very closely and monitor them for ad-verse effects. Prescribers evaluate the reported effects to determine if the causes are the diseases or the drugs. This information is collected by the drug companies developing the drugs and shared with the Food and Drug Administration. When the drugs are used widely, totally unexpected re-sponses may occur. Drugs that produce unacceptable adverse effects or unforeseen reactions are usually removed from further study.

Unacceptable adverse effects

In the past, some drugs-in-development have moved to the next stage of testing despite unacceptable effects. For example, the hypertensive drug minoxidil (Loniten) effectively treats malignant hypertension, but causes unusual hair growth on the palms and other body areas. However, because it was much more effective with the adverse effects during its development than were other antihypertensive drugs (its adverse effects not being life-threatening), it was allowed to proceed through the testing process. A few years after it was approved to treat hypertension, its hair-growing effect was channeled for therapeutic use into various hair-growth preparations such as Rogaine.

therapeutic and adverse effects. Clinical trials involve testing potential drugs on increasing numbers of human subjects. (See *Phases of clinical trials.*)

At the end of phase III studies, the data from all of the study phases are reviewed by FDA experts to determine if the drugs are effective and safe and can provide therapeutic outcomes for patients. When the FDA issues an approval letter for a drug, it includes the approved brand or proprietary name of the drug, the approved indications and dosages, all warnings, and precautions that must accompany that drug therapy.

These phases of study may reveal that certain chemicals don't bring about the desired effect, have many unacceptable adverse effects, have very small margins of safety, or are effective in only very small numbers of clinical situations. In these cases, the drugs are usually dropped from consideration and development. (See *Unacceptable adverse effects.*)

When a drug is actually on the market, it has reached phase IV, which involves the continual sur-

Consumer protection

Phase IV, or the study of drugs in widespread clinical practice after approval by the Food and Drug Administration, has been effective in protecting the public from unanticipated problems. For instance, in 1998, the antihypertensive drug mibefradil (Posicor) was removed from the market not long after its release because patients taking it had increased cardiac morbidity. In 1997, the diet drug dexfenfluramine (Redux) was removed from the market only months after its release because patients taking it developed serious heart problems. These problems weren't seen in any of the premarketing studies. Sometimes, the phase IV information can benefit patients in other ways. For example, patients taking the antiparkinsonism drug amantadine (Symmetrel) had fewer cases of influenza than other patients, leading to the discovery that amantadine is an effective antiviral agent—an attribute that wasn't noted in previous studies.

veillance of the drug's effects while it's being widely used in practice. (See *Consumer protection*.) MedWatch, a section of the FDA, collects information on adverse effects, unexpected responses, and other problems that may occur with drugs after they have been marketed. (See *Reporting problems to the FDA*.)

It takes several years and millions of dollars to take a chemical through the drug approval process. The length of time it takes has been labeled the "drug lag" because many drugs that are unavailable in the United States are in widespread use across other countries.

Generic and brand name drugs

When a company first applies to the FDA to initiate the steps to investigate a drug, an official generic name is given to its particular chemical composition. When a drug receives approval for marketing, the drug formula, much like an invention, is given a time-limited patent. The length of time that a company may hold

Reporting problems to the FDA

Even large, well-designed clinical trials can't guarantee that adverse reactions will never arise if a drug or medical device is approved for use. An adverse reaction that occurs in only 1 in 5,000 patients could easily be missed in clinical trials, but appear when hundreds of thousands of patients take the drug. The drug could also interact with other drugs in ways that are undetected during clinical trials.

As a nurse, you play a key role in reporting adverse events and other product problems. Reporting such problems helps ensure the safety of products that the Food and Drug Administration (FDA) regulates. The FDA's Medical Products Reporting Program supplies health care professionals with MedWatch forms for reporting adverse events and product problems.

WHAT TO REPORT

Complete a MedWatch form when you suspect that a drug, medical device, special nutritional product, or other product regulated by the FDA is responsible for:

✦ death
✦ life-threatening illness
✦ initial or prolonged hospitalization
✦ disability
✦ congenital anomaly
✦ need for medical or surgical intervention to prevent a permanent impairment or injury.

Also, promptly inform the FDA of product quality problems, such as:

✦ defective devices
✦ inaccurate or unreadable product labels
✦ packaging or product mix-ups
✦ intrinsic or extrinsic contamination or stability problems
✦ particulates in injectable drugs
✦ product damage.

YOUR RESPONSIBILITY IN REPORTING

When filling out a MedWatch form, keep in mind that you aren't expected to establish a connection between the product and the problem. You don't

(continued)

Reporting problems to the FDA *(continued)*

have to include a lot of details; you only have to report the adverse event or the problem with the drug or product.

What's more, don't delay reporting until the evidence seems compelling. FDA regulations protect your identity and the identities of your patient and employer.

FURTHER GUIDELINES

The MedWatch form merges the individual forms used in the past to report adverse drug reactions, drug quality problems, adverse reactions to medical devices, and medical device quality problems. Send completed forms to the FDA by using the fax number or mailing address on the form.

File a separate MedWatch form for each patient, and attach additional pages if needed. If appropriate, report product problems to the manufacturer as well as to the FDA. Also, remember to comply with your health care facility's protocols for reporting adverse events associated with drugs and medical devices.

Retain a copy of the report and the product lot number for your supervisor to keep on file. Product lot numbers are used in product identification, tracking, and recall.

FDA RESPONSE

The FDA will report back to you on the actions it takes and will continue to work to instruct health care professionals about adverse events.

the patent is determined by the chemical composition of the drug. While the patent is in effect, the company that developed the drug has the sole right to sell that drug and markets it under a specific brand or proprietary name.

MEDWATCH

THE FDA MEDICAL PRODUCTS REPORTING PROGRAM

For VOLUNTARY reporting by health professionals of adverse events and product problems

Page ___ of ___

Form Approved: OMB No. 0910-0291 Expires: 4/30/96
See OMB statement on reverse

FDA Use Only
Triage unit sequence #

A. Patient information

1. Patient identifier
2. Age at time of event:
   or —
   Date of birth:
   In confidence
3. Sex
   ☐ female
   ☐ male
4. Weight
   ___ lbs
   or
   ___ kgs

B. Adverse event or product problem

1. ☐ Adverse event and/or ☐ Product problem (e.g., defects/malfunctions)
2. Outcomes attributed to adverse event (check all that apply)
   ☐ death _____ (mo/day/yr)
   ☐ life-threatening
   ☐ hospitalization – initial or prolonged
   ☐ disability
   ☐ congenital anomaly
   ☐ required intervention to prevent permanent impairment/damage
   ☐ other:
3. Date of event (mo/day/yr)
4. Date of this report (mo/day/yr)
5. Describe event or problem

6. Relevant tests/laboratory data, including dates

7. Other relevant history, including preexisting medical conditions (e.g., allergies, race, pregnancy, smoking and alcohol use, hepatic/renal dysfunction, etc.)

PLEASE TYPE OR USE BLACK INK

C. Suspect medication(s)

1. Name (give labeled strength & mfr/labeler, if known)
   #1
   #2
2. Dose, frequency & route used
   #1
   #2
3. Therapy dates (if unknown, give duration) from/to (or best estimate)
   #1
   #2
4. Diagnosis for use (indication)
   #1
   #2
5. Event abated after use stopped or dose reduced
   #1 ☐ yes ☐ no ☐ doesn't apply
   #2 ☐ yes ☐ no ☐ doesn't apply
6. Lot # (if known)
   #1
   #2
7. Exp. date (if known)
   #1
   #2
8. Event reappeared after reintroduction
   #1 ☐ yes ☐ no ☐ doesn't apply
   #2 ☐ yes ☐ no ☐ doesn't apply
9. NDC # (for product problems only)
10. Concomitant medical products and therapy dates (exclude treatment of event)

D. Suspect medical device

1. Brand name
2. Type of device
3. Manufacturer name & address
4. Operator of device
   ☐ health professional
   ☐ lay user/patient
   ☐ other:
5. Expiration date (mo/day/yr)
6. model # _____
   catalog # _____
   serial # _____
   lot # _____
   other # _____
7. If implanted, give date (mo/day/yr)
8. If explanted, give date (mo/day/yr)
9. Device available for evaluation? (Do not send to FDA)
   ☐ yes ☐ no ☐ returned to manufacturer on _____ (mo/day/yr)
10. Concomitant medical products and therapy dates (exclude treatment of event)

E. Reporter (see confidentiality section on back)

1. Name & address   phone #
2. Health professional? ☐ yes ☐ no
3. Occupation
4. Also reported to
   ☐ manufacturer
   ☐ user facility
   ☐ distributor
5. If you do NOT want your identity disclosed to the manufacturer, place an " X " in this box. ☐

FDA

Mail to: MEDWATCH
5600 Fishers Lane
Rockville, MD 20852-9787
or FAX to: 1-800-FDA-0178

FDA Form 3500 (1/96)   Submission of a report does not constitute an admission that medical personnel or the product caused or contributed to the event.

For example, Prozac is the brand name for the popular antidepressant known generically as fluoxetine. In August 2001, the patent expired on fluoxetine, allowing other manufacturers to produce the drug. Although these other companies can't use the name

Problems with generic drugs

In the past, some quality control issues with generic products have created problems. For example, the binders used in a generic drug may not be the same as those used in the brand name product, so the way the body breaks down and uses the generic drug (the drug's bioavailability) may differ from that of the brand name product.

Many states and insurers require that a drug be dispensed in the generic form if one is available. This requirement is intended to keep down drugs' cost.

Some prescribers, however, request that a drug be "dispensed as written"—that is, the brand name product be used. By doing this, the prescriber ensures the quality control and bioavailability expected with that drug. These concerns may be most important in drugs that have narrow safety margins, such as digoxin (Lanoxin) and warfarin (Coumadin). If a patient has taken a specific drug for a long time and suddenly no longer responds to the drug or develops other effects, it's important to check if the patient was switched to a generic form.

Prozac, they can sell the drug under the generic name fluoxetine.

Companies that produce generic drugs don't have the research, advertising or, sometimes, the quality control departments that pharmaceutical companies have. Usually, this allows them to produce the generic drugs more cheaply. However, because the bioavailability of the generic drugs may differ from that of proprietary drugs due to quality control problems, some prescribers may specify a brand-name drug despite state requirements for prescribing generic drugs when available. (See *Problems with generic drugs*.)

Orphan drugs
Orphan drugs refer to those compounds that progress through the approval process, but because they

weren't financially viable, fail to be "adopted" by a drug company.

Orphan drugs may be useful in treating only a rare disease. For example, many orphan drugs are used to treat rare neuromuscular diseases or cancers, but because the number of people with these disorders is so small, the projected sales of the drug don't come close to covering the expense of the approval process. Also, some orphan drugs have potentially dangerous adverse effects or have such a small margin of safety that the drug companies that developed them would need to be concerned about potential lawsuits and the public's welfare.

The Orphan Drug Act of 1983 provides tremendous financial incentives to drug companies to adopt and develop these drugs. When an orphan drug use is listed for a particular disorder, it means that it was found to be effective for treating that disorder, but the financial risks are too great for the drug company. Because of the potential value of the drug to certain patients, the government offers the drug company tax relief to develop it for approved usage.

Over-the-counter drugs

Products that are available without prescriptions for self-treatment of various complaints are called "over-the-counter" (OTC) drugs. Some of these drugs have never gone through the rigorous testing that's now required for drug approval, but were "grandfathered" into use when the more stringent laws were passed because they had already been used for so long. Aspirin is one such drug.

Other drugs were originally approved for prescription use only, but over time were released as OTCs. Research found them to be safe and effective for consumer self-administration, as directed on packaging.

Problems with over-the-counter drugs

Patients may not even consider over-the-counter (OTC) drugs to be medications and commonly don't report using them. People frequently look only at the advertisement or picture on the box and don't try to read or understand what the ingredients are or what warnings might be attached to the drug.

Some patients don't even read the dosing instructions. "If one makes me feel better, two will make me feel really good" isn't always a safe approach when using these drugs. The overall impression people have of OTC drugs is that if you can buy them without a prescription, they must be safe.

Because of the potential impact of OTC drugs on a diagnosis or a drug regimen, nurses should always include specific questions about OTC drug use when taking a patient's drug history. It's also very important that all drug-teaching protocols provide information about avoiding OTC drugs when taking prescription drugs, or at least checking with a health care provider before choosing and using an OTC drug.

Frequently, the OTC recommended dosage is less than the recommended prescription dosage.

Although OTC drugs have been found to be safe when "taken as directed," there are several problems related to OTC drugs.

✦ Taking these drugs may mask the signs and symptoms of underlying disease, making diagnosis difficult.

✦ Taking these drugs with prescription medications may result in drug interactions and can interfere with drug therapy.

✦ Not taking these drugs "as directed" may result in serious overdoses. (See *Problems with over-the-counter drugs.*)

Legal regulation of drugs

The FDA regulates the development and sale of drugs. Local laws further regulate the distribution and administration of drugs. In most cases, the strictest law prevails. Nurses should become familiar with the rules and regulations in the areas in which they practice. These regulations may vary from state to state, and many even vary within states. Ignorance isn't an excuse in legal matters, and nurses should be aware of not only their facility's policies, but also of the local state laws that affect practice.

Pregnancy categories

As part of the standards for testing and safety, the FDA requires that each new drug be assigned a pregnancy category. The categories indicate a drug's potential or actual adverse effects on the fetus, called teratogenic effects, thus offering guidelines for use of a particular drug during pregnancy. (See *FDA pregnancy categories,* page 16.)

Research into the development of the human fetus, especially its nervous system, has led many health care providers to recommend that no drug be used during pregnancy because of potential effects on the developing fetus. In cases in which a drug is needed, it's recommended that the drug of choice should be that for which the benefit clearly outweighs the potential risks.

Controlled substances

The Controlled Substances Act of 1970 establishes categories of rank for potentially abusive drugs. This same act gives control over the coding of drugs and the enforcement of these codes to the FDA and the Drug Enforcement Agency (DEA), a part of the Department of Justice. The FDA studies the drugs and determines their abuse potential; the DEA enforces their control. Drugs with abuse potential are called controlled sub-

FDA pregnancy categories

The Food and Drug Administration (FDA) has established five categories to indicate the potential for a systemically absorbed drug to cause birth defects. The key differentiation among the categories rests upon the degree and reliability of documentation and the risk-benefit ratio. Regardless of its designated pregnancy category or presumed safety, no drug should be administered during pregnancy unless the mother clearly needs it.

CATEGORY A

Adequate studies in pregnant women haven't demonstrated a risk to the fetus in the first trimester of pregnancy, and there's no evidence of risk in later trimesters.

CATEGORY B

Animal studies haven't demonstrated a risk to the fetus, but there are no adequate studies in pregnant women. Or, although animal studies have shown an adverse effect, adequate studies in pregnant women haven't demonstrated a risk to the fetus during the first trimester of pregnancy, and there's no evidence of risk in later trimesters.

CATEGORY C

Animal studies have shown an adverse effect on the fetus, but there are no adequate studies in humans; the benefits from the use of the drug in pregnant women may be acceptable despite potential risks. Or, there are no animal studies and no adequate studies in humans.

CATEGORY D

There's evidence of human fetal risk, but the potential benefits from using the drug in pregnant women may be acceptable despite potential risks.

CATEGORY X

Studies in animals or humans demonstrate fetal abnormalities or adverse reactions; reports indicate evidence of fetal risk. The risk of use in a pregnant woman clearly outweighs a possible benefit.

Controlled substance schedules

Controlled drugs are divided into five Drug Enforcement Agency (DEA) schedules based on their potential for physical and psychological dependence and abuse. Prescribers and dispensing pharmacists must be registered with the DEA, which also provides forms for the transfer of schedule I and II substances and establishes criteria for the inventory and prescribing of controlled substances. State and local laws are commonly more stringent than federal law. In any given situation, the more stringent law applies.

Schedule I (C-I): High abuse potential and no accepted medical use (heroin, marijuana, and LSD).

Schedule II (C-II): High abuse potential with severe dependence liability (narcotics, amphetamines, and barbiturates).

Schedule III (C-III): Less abuse potential than schedule II drugs, and moderate dependence liability (nonbarbiturate sedatives, nonamphetamine stimulants, and limited amounts of certain narcotics).

Schedule IV (C-IV): Less abuse potential than schedule III drugs and limited dependence liability (some sedatives, antianxiety agents, and nonnarcotic analgesics).

Schedule V (C-V): Limited abuse potential (primarily small amounts of narcotics, such as codeine, used as antitussives or antidiarrheals). Under federal law, limited quantities of certain schedule V drugs may be purchased without a prescription directly from a pharmacist. The purchaser must be at least age 18 and must furnish suitable identification. The dispensing pharmacist must record all such transactions.

stances. The prescription, distribution, storage, and use of these drugs are closely monitored by the DEA to decrease their abuse. Each prescriber has a DEA number, which allows the agency to monitor prescription patterns and possible abuse. (See *Controlled substance schedules*.)

A nurse should be familiar with DEA guidelines for controlled substances as well as local policies and procedures, which might be more rigorous. Storage and administration policies for controlled substances vary widely among states, facilities, and units within facilities. It's the nurse's responsibility to become familiar with the policies in force in a specific clinical setting. As with other laws, the more stringent law prevails if legal problems occur.

Laws affecting drug administration

State laws regulate the preparation and dispensing of drugs (in most states, the role of the pharmacist), the prescription of a drug (the role of the physician, physician assistant, or nurse practitioner), and the administration of a drug (in most states, the role of the nurse).

PREVENT IT

Medication error: Even back in 1944, practice limits were the subject of legal cases. In a case in Rhode Island— Stefanik v. Nursing Education Committee *— a nurse lost her license because she changed a physician's order when she didn't agree with what he had prescribed. The patient wasn't harmed, but the Nurse Practice Act of Rhode Island clearly stated that a nurse can't prescribe medications. Changing the order was considered to be the same as writing an order for a new drug.*

Prevention: Many times in practice, a nurse may question or disagree with a medication order. Communication is the best approach. Discuss your concerns, listen to the rationale and, if you still strongly disagree, refuse to give the drug and ask someone else or the prescriber to administer the drug. You're responsible for your own actions.

The Nurse Practice Act of each state defines the tasks that belong to the nurse in that state. It also states that anyone who performs these tasks without a license is breaking the law. In many states, except for a specially licensed nurse practitioner, a nurse who prescribes drugs or goes into a drug storage area and measures a drug dose would be considered practicing pharmacy without a license. In many situations, these legal errors would be misdemeanors at best, and in other situations could cost the nurse her license.

In various medical environments, it's common practice for nurses to have the responsibility for checking drug dosage calculations, proper storage of drugs, and assuring that the narcotic drug count balances—narcotics dispensed versus narcotics available. Hopefully, the facility's policies concerning these actions were established with guidance from the legislation that governs the Nurse Practice Act.

It's important for nurses to be aware of federal, state, and local policies when practicing nursing. If an emergency situation, such as a severe shortage of nurses and pharmacists, or another factor results in a policy that's contradictory with your understanding of the law, get the legal facts. Even when a staffing shortage has led to "acceptable" shortcuts in your particular situation, you can still lose your license if you violate existing laws.

PREVENT IT

Medication error: In 1981, in the case of Sessauer v. Memorial General Hospital *in New Mexico, a family won a lawsuit against a hospital whose staffing problems resulted in medication errors. An obstetric nurse was floated to the emergency department (ED) because of a staffing shortage and a busy ED. The nurse gave a patient 800 mg of lidocaine when the ED physician had ordered 50 mg. The patient died. The nurse was unfamiliar with emergency medicine and the usual drugs and dosages used in that setting. The court concluded that was no excuse for the error.*

Prevention: *Although the nurse was under strain and out of her usual area of expertise, she should have questioned any drug she was asked to give. The error could have been prevented if the nurse simply explained that she was unfamiliar with emergency medicine and asked that the order be repeated or clarified—a request that should have been respected by the staff.*

Off-label uses of drugs

When the FDA approves a drug, its approval extends only to clearly stated therapeutic indications. These approved indications reflect the research carried out on the drug and the balance of benefit versus risk and adverse effects associated with the drug. After a drug is available, however, it's often used for indications for which it hasn't been approved. This "off-label" use is very common in patient populations for whom little premarketing testing has been done—especially pediatric and geriatric populations. Given the ethical issues involved in testing drugs on children, many drugs go to market with only adult indications, having not been tested for use in children. The use of a particular drug in children often occurs as trial and error after the drug is released without pediatric indications or nursing considerations. Thus, dosing calculations and nomograms become very important in determining the approximate dose that should be used for a child.

Drugs are also used for various psychiatric disorders for which they haven't been approved. Because little is really known about the way the brain works and what happens when the chemicals in the brain are altered, a

polypharmacy approach in psychiatry has occurred—
mixing and juggling drugs until the desired effect is
achieved. A combination that works for one patient
might not work for another patient with the same diagnosis because of brain and chemical differences in that
patient.

Off-label use is widespread and may lead to the discovery of a new use for a drug. However, nurses need to be
aware that the liability issues surrounding off-label uses
are unclear. You should be clear about a drug's intended
use, why it's being tried, and the potential for problems. If
you have doubts about the use of a particular drug for a
given problem, verify the accuracy of the prescription.
When in doubt, always "check it out" with a drug reference text, supervisor, pharmacist, or the prescriber.

Alternative therapies and herbal medicine

Other drugs that the practicing nurse needs to be aware
of are the growing and increasingly popular herbal therapies. Referenced in ancient records, these drugs are commonly the basis for the discovery of an active ingredient
that has been successfully developed into a modern regulated medication. These drugs are made from ground
roots, leaves, flowers, bark, or even seeds from a variety
of plants found in nature.

These products and their active ingredients aren't controlled or tested by the FDA. The Dietary Supplement
Health and Education Act of 1994, updated in 2000,
states that herbal products as well as vitamins, minerals,
and amino acids are classified as dietary supplements and
aren't required to go through extensive premarketing
testing.

Numerous Web sites tout natural treatments that consumers can use to cure many disorders without ever having to see their health care providers. Many people who
want to gain control of their medical care or who don't

want to take "drugs" for their diabetes, depression, arthritis, or fatigue are drawn to these products.

Advertising of herbal and alternative therapies isn't as restricted or accurate as that of classic drugs. In television or magazine ads, consumers are urged to use the "natural" approach to medical care and self-treat with a wide variety of products. Advertisements for these products aren't permitted to make direct claims to cure, treat, diagnose, or prevent a specific disease, but may make nondisease claims, such as "for muscle enhancement," "for hot flashes," or "for memory loss." Disclaimers reveal that these products aren't tested or approved by the FDA and that they aren't intended to treat or cure disease, but they're flashed quickly to deter viewer comprehension. Packaging disclaimers, minutely printed, are lost among eye-catching graphics.

Alternative therapies are unregulated, poorly understood, typically used without the knowledge or guidance of health care providers, and have the potential to interact with each other and with prescribed drugs. Consequently, they may contribute to undesirable actions and adverse effects and are perceived as actual medication errors. The nursing assessment must always include all prescribed and OTC drugs as well as any herbal or alternative therapies the patient is using. (See *Problems with alternative therapies.*)

PREVENT IT

Medication error: *D.C., a 46-year-old sales representative, was diagnosed with type 2 diabetes. Her condition was stabilized with diet, exercise, and glipizide. She had lost several family members to complications of diabetes and was very diligent about following her diet, exercise, and medication plan. About 10 months after her diagnosis, she was seen in*

Problems with alternative therapies

Health care providers need to be concerned with several issues when a patient elects to self-treat with herbal and other alternative therapies.

VARIABLE EFFECTS

Active ingredients in alternative products haven't been tested by the Food and Drug Administration or they may have been tested on only very few people with no reproducible results. For example, when a patient takes bilberry to control diabetes, the reaction is unpredictable. In some patients, blood glucose may fall; in others it may rise.

PRODUCT ADDITIVES

Incidental ingredients in many alternative products are unknown. Because most of these products are produced directly from plants or from a natural, unchemically altered state, their efficacy may be influenced by the fertilizer used on the plant, the time of year the plant is harvested, and other ingredients the manufacturer compounds with the plant.

For example, saw palmetto, an herb used to alleviate the symptoms of benign prostatic hypertrophy, is available in several preparations from different manufacturers. A random sampling of these products, performed in 2000, found that the amount of the identified active ingredient varied from 20% to 400% of the recommended dose. With such a wide range of variability, guiding patients to the correct product is difficult.

CONCOMITANT USE

Patients commonly don't mention the use of alternative therapies to their health care providers. Some patients feel that their provider wouldn't approve of the use and don't wish to discuss it. Additionally, others feel that these are just natural products and don't need to be mentioned. However, with increasing use of these products have come reports of drug interactions that can cause serious complications for patients who are taking prescription medications.

For example, patients with diabetes who decide to use juniper berries, ginseng, garlic, fenugreek, coriander, dandelion root, or celery to "help maintain their blood glucose level" may experience serious problems with hypoglycemia when they also use their prescription diabetic drugs. If the pa-

(continued)

Problems with alternative therapies *(continued)*

tients don't report the use of these alternative therapies to their health care provider, they may undergo extensive medical tests and dosage adjustments to no avail.

St. John's wort, a highly advertised and popular alternative therapy for depression, has been found to interact with oral contraceptives, digoxin, selective serotonin reuptake inhibitors, and the antivirals used in treating acquired immunodeficiency syndrome. Patients using St. John's wort along with Prozac for the symptoms of depression may experience serious adverse effects and toxic reactions. If health care providers don't know about the use of St. John's wort, treating the toxicity can become very complicated.

It's important to ask the patient specifically about the use of herbal or alternative treatment products. This should become a routine part of the health history and is particularly important if the patient presents with an unexpected reaction to a medication.

the clinic following 3 days of hypoglycemia that she wasn't able to regulate with eating. She stated that she felt dizzy, fatigued, weak, and anxious. She reported that she hadn't taken other medications, had been following her protocol religiously, and hadn't had stressors in her life. She was stabilized in the clinic. While following D.C.'s progress, the nurse found out that D.C. had become very interested in nutritional and herbal therapy following a walk through the mall. She had been counseled by the sales representative at a nutritional center and had been using ginseng, garlic, astragalus, and juniper berry tea. After researching these products, the nurse discovered that they all contribute to lowering blood sugar and had compounded the effect of her prescribed regimen to produce D.C.'s current medical problem.

Prevention: This problem could have been avoided if D.C. had been cautioned during her initial diabetic teaching program to report the use of herbal or alternative treatment *products. She could use herbal supplements as long as the dosage and timing of her other prescribed medication was considered in the total regimen. Diabetic control can be very fragile, and many herbal products are known to interfere with glucose levels in the body. The patient with diabetes should always be cautioned to report and discuss the use of these products with her health care provider.*

✦ Changes in health care

The cost of medical care and drugs has exploded in the past few years. In part, this stems from consumer demand to have the best possible, most up-to-date, and safest drug care therapies available. At the same time, the rising cost of health insurance to pay for this care is a major complaint of employers and consumers. As a result, health maintenance organizations (HMOs) have surged in popularity. These groups run the medical care system like a business, with the financial aspects commonly becoming the overriding concern and decisions being made by nonmedical personnel with a keen eye on the bottom line. Patients are being discharged from hospitals much earlier than they once were — supposedly a cost-saving move. Many more aren't even admitted to hospitals for surgical or invasive procedures that once required several days of hospital care and monitoring by nurses.

The result is less direct nursing care and monitoring of patients, with responsibility for self-care and monitoring falling to the patient or caregiver. Teaching the patient about self-care, drug therapies, and what to expect is more crucial now than ever, and it's the nurse who's usually responsible for this education.

Special drug therapy concerns

HMOs may regulate access to emergency facilities, types and timing of tests allowed, procedures covered, and prescription drugs. The formulary for each HMO differs. Sometimes only generic products are covered, and the patient must pay for newer drugs. In other cases, there's a tier system of costs, and the patient may urge the prescriber to choose a drug from a lower tier at a lower cost. Many health care providers believe that their ability to make decisions is limited by regulations and that decisions are commonly made by nonmedical personnel who have no contact with the patient. The regulatory power of HMOs is being challenged in various court cases and through legislation and may change dramatically in the future. It's important for patients to check rules and guidelines for their particular medical coverage as each case may be unique.

Cost considerations

It's usually necessary for the health care provider to choose drug therapy based on the cost of the drugs available and the insurance a patient may have for prescription medications. With more of the population reaching retirement age and depending on a fixed income, cost can be a significant issue. Sometimes, this may mean not selecting a first-choice drug but settling for one that should be effective.

The nurse can teach the patient nondrug methods to enhance the drug therapy regimen prescribed. For example, in an effort to save money, some patients may stop taking antibiotics after they feel better, saving the rest for the next time they feel sick. This practice has helped to contribute to the problem of resistant bacteria, which is becoming more dangerous. The nurse needs to teach the patient to take the full course of antibiotics and not stop the drug when they feel better.

In addition, nurses should advise patients not to cut tablets in half unless specifically instructed to do so. Patients sometimes perceive that cutting tablets in half affords them twice the drug therapy. Others feel they won't become dependent on a drug if they take half the prescribed dose and still have it work effectively. However, some drugs must not be cut. With the new matrix delivery systems used in many drugs, cutting the drug may cause toxicity or decrease its effectiveness. The cost of treating the toxic reactions may far exceed the cost of the original drug.

Home care safety issues

The home care industry is one of the most rapidly expanding areas in health care, its growth fueled by the changes in costs and the delivery of medical care. Because insurance companies limit hospital stays based on practice diagnoses, patients go home directly from surgery with the responsibility for changing dressings, assessing wounds, managing drug regimens, and monitoring their own rehabilitation and recovery. At the same time, the population is aging and some patients may be less accepting or capable of these responsibilities. As a result, some health aides, visiting nurses, and home care programs are taking over some of the responsibilities that were previously handled in the hospital. Consequently, discharge patient education has increased astronomically in the past decade, and nurses are responsible for most if not all patient teaching. Moreover, the nurse must initiate discharge planning and teaching during the admission process.

Patients need to know exactly what medications they're taking (generic and brand names), the dosages of those medications, and how and when they're supposed to take them. Patients also need to know what they can do to alleviate some of the adverse effects expected with each drug, what OTC or alternative therapies they need to avoid while taking each drug, and what specific signs or symptoms to report to their health care provider. For patients taking multiple drugs at the same time, this information should be provided in writing with language that's clear and understandable.

Many pharmacies provide printouts of information with each drug dispensed. However, in many instances the information is incomprehensible to the lay person, and the information is too abundant and confusing to organize if the patient is taking multiple drugs. During patient-teaching sessions, the nurse organizes, simplifies, and helps the patient understand the information given to him by the pharmacist. Having nurses educate patients about their drug therapy increases patient safety and reduces costs related to treating adverse effects.

The cost of incomplete patient teaching is high. Dealing with toxic or adverse effects is usually more costly than taking time to fully educate the patient. The projections for trends in health care indicate a greater expansion of the home health care system, with hospitals being used for only the most critically ill patients. The nurse's role in this home health system — as teacher, assessor, problem solver, and patient advocate — is increasingly crucial.

Chapter

The nurse's role in drug management

The delivery of medical care today is in a constant state of change. The population is aging, resulting in more chronic disease and complex care issues. The population also is transient, resulting in unstable support systems and fewer at-home care providers and helpers. At the same time, medicine is undergoing a technological boom — computed tomography scans, nuclear magnetic resonance imaging, experimental drugs. These changes are affecting the rate, type, and place of patient care. Patients are being discharged earlier from acute care facilities or aren't being admitted at all for procedures that used to be treated in-hospital with follow-up support and monitoring. Patients are becoming more responsible for their own care and for following complicated medical regimens at home.

✦ Nursing: Art and science

Nursing is a unique and complex science as well as a nurturing and caring art. Traditionally, nursing has been viewed as ministering to and soothing the sick. In the current state of health care, nursing also has become increasingly technical and scientific. Nurses have had to assume increasing responsibilities that involve not only nurturing and caring, but also assessing, problem identifying, and intervening with patients to treat, prevent, and educate them to cope with various health states.

The nurse deals with the whole person: the physical, emotional, intellectual, social, and spiritual. She needs to consider how a person responds to disease, treatment, and the change in lifestyle that may be required for health. The nurse is the key health care provider who's in the position to assess the whole patient; administer therapy, including medications; teach the patient how to best cope with therapy to assure the best outcomes; and evaluate the effectiveness of the therapy. To do all this, the nurse must have a broad knowledge base in the basic sciences (anatomy, physiology, nutrition, chemistry, pharmacology), the social sciences (sociology, psychology), education, and other disciplines.

✦ The nursing process

Although all nursing theorists don't agree on the process that defines nursing practice, most agree upon certain key elements. These elements are the basic components of the decision-making or problem-solving process:

- ✦ assessment: gathering information
- ✦ nursing diagnosis: analyzing the information gathered to arrive at a conclusion
- ✦ clinical intervention: taking action to meet the patient's needs, such as administering drugs or therapies, teaching, and providing comfort measures
- ✦ evaluation: determining the effects of the interventions performed.

The nursing process provides the nurse with an organized and comprehensive method of approaching each clinical situation. Without an organized approach, many situations may seem completely overwhelming.

With respect to drug therapy, the nursing process ensures that the patient receives the best, most efficient, and safest care possible.

Assessment

The first step of the problem-solving process is always the systematic, organized collection of data. Because nurses are responsible for holistic care of a patient, these data must include details about physical, intellectual, emotional, social, and environmental factors. This information provides the facts needed to plan teaching and discharge programs, arrange for appropriate consultations, and monitor a disease process or a patient's response to drug therapy.

In clinical practice, because the patient isn't static, the actual assessment process never ends. The patient is in a dynamic state, adjusting to physical, emotional, and environmental influences, sometimes on a minute-to-minute basis. With experience, each nurse develops a unique approach to organizing the assessment, an approach that's functional and useful in the clinical setting and that makes sense to that nurse and the given situation. A nurse who works in a cardiac intensive care unit (CICU) may become quite adept at assessing cardiovascular factors, whereas one who works in a dermatology clinic may often assess cardiovascular factors but may more efficiently assess the skin and related structures. A nurse who works on a busy surgical floor may seem to respond reflexively when a patient vomits, falls and rips out staples, or begins bleeding profusely. With heightened awareness of the events that could occur in that setting, that nurse adopts an assessment process that permits quick evaluation. That same nurse may not react as efficiently if she were asked to work in the CICU because the assessment needs are different. The process of each area of nursing practice isn't overwhelming to nurses who work in that area; rather, it becomes second nature.

Drug therapy is a complex and important part of most health care, and the principles of drug therapy need to be incorporated into every patient assessment plan. Although the particular information that needs to be assessed varies with each drug, the concepts involved are similar. Two key areas that always need to be assessed are the patient's history and his physical status.

Patient history

The patient's past experiences and illnesses can influence a drug's effect.

Chronic conditions

The presence of certain conditions, such as renal disease, heart disease, diabetes, and chronic lung disease, may contraindicate the use of a drug, require that caution be used when administering a certain drug, or indicate that the drug dosage needs to be adjusted. For example, the use of aspirin would be contraindicated in a patient with chronic renal failure.

Drug use

Prescription drugs, over-the-counter (OTC) drugs, street drugs, alcohol, nicotine, alternative therapies such as herbs and vitamins, and caffeine may have an impact on a drug's effect. Some of these drugs may increase the toxicity of prescription drugs, whereas others may block their effects. Ask patients specifically about their use of OTC drugs, alternative therapies, and prescription drugs. They commonly neglect to mention OTC drugs or alternative therapies, not thinking of them as drugs or not willing to admit to their health care provider that they use them. When giving a drug history, a patient commonly fails to mention taking oral contraceptives, replacement therapies (such as thyroid hormone), or other drugs he takes daily because these drugs have become part of the daily routine and the patient doesn't even think about them.

Allergies

Past reactions to a drug or other allergens can predict a future reaction or note a caution for the use of a drug, food, or animal product. It's important to have the patient describe the allergic reaction when reporting a drug allergy. In some cases, the reaction isn't an allergic response but an actual drug effect or adverse reaction.

Level of education

Information about a patient's education level helps you determine the level of explanation required and amount of understanding expected. It also provides a basis for developing an effective patient-teaching program. Assessing the patient's understanding of his disease and therapy also helps you develop appropriate educational information and discharge planning.

Social supports

Patients, who are now being discharged earlier than they were in the past, often need help at home with care and management of drug therapy. A key aspect of discharge planning involves determining what support, if any, is available to patients at home. In many situations, discharge planning also involves referral to appropriate community resources.

Financial supports

The high cost of health care in general, and of medications in particular, needs to be considered when initiating drug therapy. Because of financial constraints, a patient may not follow through with the prescribed regimen for an expensive drug. In some situations, a less costly drug might adequately replace a more expensive one. In such cases, you may refer the patient to appropriate sources for financial assistance.

Pattern of health care
Knowing how a patient seeks health care gives you valuable information to include in your teaching plan. Does this patient routinely seek follow-up care or wait for emergency situations? Does the patient tend to self-treat many complaints or bring every problem to a health care provider?

Having this information handy helps you prepare written information for drug therapy or discharge planning. Some patients need strict schedules and appointment outlines; others need to feel some control over their situations and want to have input into decisions and treatment regimens.

Physical status
The patient's physical status is important when determining the appropriate use of certain drugs. It also provides the baseline information needed to evaluate the patient's response to drug therapy. Although the patient's diagnosis and the anticipated effects of the intended drug determine the actual parameters you must assess, certain factors influence drug therapy. (See *Key history points*.)

Weight
A patient's weight helps determine whether the recommended drug dosage is appropriate. Because the recommended dosage typically is calculated for a 150 lb (68 kg) adult male, patients who are much lighter or much heavier may need an adjusted dosage.

Age
Patients at the extremes of the age spectrum — children and older adults — commonly require adjusted

---

✦

Key history points

When taking the patient's history, be sure to ask about:
+ chronic conditions
+ drug use
  - prescription drugs
  - over-the-counter drugs
  - herbal therapies
  - street drugs
  - nicotine, caffeine, alcohol
+ allergies: drug and reaction
+ level of education
+ understanding of medical condition and therapy
+ social supports
+ financial supports
+ pattern of health care
+ physical assessment:
  - weight
  - age
  - physical parameters related to disease state or known
drug therapy.

---

dosages based on the functional level of the liver and kidneys and the responsiveness of other organs. Women of childbearing age should always be questioned about the possibility of pregnancy before a drug is given.

Physical parameters related to the disease state or known drug effects

Assessing physical factors before beginning drug therapy provides a baseline for comparing future assessments to determine the effects of drug therapy. The specific parameters that need to be assessed depend on the patient's disease process and on the expected therapeutic and adverse effects of the drug therapy.

For example, if a patient is being treated for chronic pulmonary disease, respiratory status and reserve need to be assessed, especially if a drug is being given that has known effects on the respiratory tract. In contrast, a thorough respiratory evaluation isn't warranted in a patient who doesn't have pulmonary disease and who's taking a drug with no known effects on the respiratory system. Because you have the greatest direct and continual contact with the patient, you have the best opportunity to detect minute changes that ultimately determine the course of drug therapy — therapeutic success or discontinuation because of adverse or unacceptable responses.

Nursing diagnoses

After collecting data, you must organize and analyze it to arrive at a nursing diagnosis — a statement of a problem that the patient is experiencing or at risk for developing from a nursing perspective. This statement directs appropriate nursing interventions. A nursing diagnosis shows actual or potential alteration in patient function based on the assessment of the clinical situation. Because drug therapy is only a small part of the overall patient situation, nursing diagnoses related to drug therapy must be incorporated into a total picture of the patient.

Clinical interventions

The assessment and diagnosis of the patient directs specific nursing interventions. There are three types of interventions that are usually involved in drug therapy: drug administration, provision of comfort measures, and patient and family teaching.

Proper drug administration

There are five "rights" established for the safe and effective administration of a drug. They are:

✦ *The right patient.* This point is quite simple — check to make sure that you're giving the drug to the patient for whom it's intended. As important, make sure the patient has no allergies to that drug, isn't taking interacting drugs or alternative therapies, and has no contraindications or cautions to the use of that drug.

✦ *The right drug.* The drug to be administered must match the one the prescriber ordered. Sometimes that's a challenge; sound-alike and look-alike names have made it difficult to match the intended drug with the available drug. It's also the nurse's responsibility to make sure the drug is appropriate for that patient — does the patient have a diagnosis the drug is indicated to treat? Will this drug help, not harm, this patient? It's also important to make sure that this drug was stored properly to ensure safety (some drugs have very specific storage directions) and that it was prepared properly for administration. (Some drugs need to be diluted and some drugs can be cut or crushed, whereas others can't.)

✦ *The right dose.* In many settings, the nurse receives a unit dose product and may assume that it's the correct dose. The nurse is the last check in the system safeguards and must review the calculations and check to make sure this is actually the correct dose for this drug for the patient. Drugs have recommended dosages, but remember that those dosages were usually established for males of a certain weight. If a drug has a recommended pediatric or geriatric dosage, or a dosage for a patient with, for example, renal or hepatic dysfunction, you need to make sure the dosage ordered corresponds with these guidelines. If in doubt, check it out. However, it's also important to consider the patient's weight, physical factors that may alter the drug's effects, and use of other drugs or alternative therapies that may alter the drug levels. Sometimes the drug dosage that's needed isn't the dosage that's available, and you'll need to calculate how many tablets or milliliters are needed to deliver the desired dose. Sometimes it's also necessary to calculate drug dosage based on the patient's body weight, surface area, or renal function tests.

✦ *The right route.* Determining the best administration route is usually established by the drug's formulation — for example, some drugs are available only for injection, others are available only for inhalation. Nurses can commonly influence the modification of the route to arrive at the most efficient, comfortable delivery for the patient based on the patient's specific situation. For example, the prescriber may not know that the patient isn't able to swallow tablets and would benefit from a liquid preparation. When it's determined that the right route has been selected for this patient and this drug, it's important to make sure that route is being used effectively. Inhaled drugs are used differently than nasal sprays, and the application of an ophthalmic cream is different than applying eye drops. When in doubt, check it out. A quick review of the proper administration technique can prevent problems. This is especially important when teaching a patient the proper method of drug administration. Studies have shown that it's difficult to "unteach" the wrong technique — teaching the right technique the first time is much more effective.

✦ *The right time*. Administration of one drug may need to be coordinated with the administration of other drugs, foods, or physical parameters. The caregiver most involved in administering drugs must be aware of and balance these factors as well as educate patients to do this on their own. Patients managing their drugs at home seldom use the same time schedule as hospitals do, and it's important to help patients determine an easy way to incorporate their drug therapy into a daily routine. Patients have reported taking all of their day's medications at once, first thing in the morning, to avoid missing any doses. This can have serious ramifications if some of those drugs were intended for three-times-per-day use, or interact with other drugs, and may lead to such complications as the development of resistant strains of bacteria.

After assessing the patient, making the appropriate nursing diagnoses, and delivering the correct drug, in the correct dose, by the correct route, and at the correct time, documentation of that information in accordance with facility policy is necessary. Not only is this a legal requirement, but it's also an important reference if the patient has an unexpected drug reaction or adverse effect. In many disciplinary and legal actions, documentation is the key element; if it isn't written, it didn't happen.

Providing comfort measures

The nurse is in a unique position to help the patient cope with the effects of drug therapy. This may involve teaching the patient to incorporate the effects of a diuretic into the day's schedule or to avoid the sun if a drug causes photosensitivity. The provision of comfort measures usually falls into three main categories.

✦ *Facilitating the placebo effect.* The anticipation that a drug will have a specific effect (placebo effect) has been shown to have tremendous impact on the actual success of drug therapy. In the same way, the nurse can display a positive attitude about the outcome of a medication (for example, stating, "This will make you feel better soon" when administering a pain medication).

✦ *Managing adverse effects.* There are interventions that can decrease the impact of a drug's anticipated adverse effects and promote the patient's safety. Such interventions include teaching him about environmental control (temperature, light), safety measures (using side rails, avoiding the sun, avoiding driving), and physical comfort (skin care, laxatives, frequent meals).

✦ *Working with the patient to make lifestyle adjustments.* Some drug effects require that a patient change his lifestyle to cope effectively. For example, the patient taking a diuretic may have to rearrange the day's schedule to be near toilet facilities when the drugs take effect. The patient taking a monoamine oxidase inhibitor has to adjust his diet to prevent serious adverse effects from drug interaction with certain foods. In some cases, the necessary change in lifestyle can have a tremendous impact on the patient and affect coping and compliance with the medical regimen.

Patient and family teaching

With patients becoming increasingly responsible for their own care, it's essential that they have all the information necessary to ensure safe and effective drug therapy at home. (See *Guidelines for effective drug teaching.*) In fact, many states now require that patients be given written information about their prescriptions. The information provided to a patient or family mem-

Guidelines for effective drug teaching

When explaining a patient's drug regimen, be sure to include:

✦ the drug's name (generic and proprietary), dosage, and indication
✦ timing of administration
✦ special storage and preparation instructions
✦ over-the-counter drugs or herbal therapies to avoid
✦ specific comfort measures to use
✦ safety measures, including protecting children and reporting all drug use to other providers
✦ warnings about drug discontinuation
✦ toxicity effects to report.

ber about a specific drug varies with the drug, the route of administration, and the cautions or warnings associated with that drug.

Key elements that need to be included in a drug education program are:

✦ *Name, dose, and action of drug.* Many patients see and must communicate with more than one health care provider, so having information about all the drugs they're taking is crucial to ensuring safe and effective drug therapy and avoiding drug-drug interactions. Patients may state that they take a "heart drug" or an "asthma" drug, but with the choices available today, that may not be sufficient information with which to prevent toxicity, an overdose, or a drug-drug interaction.

✦ *Timing of administration.* Teach the patient when to take the drug in respect to frequency, other drugs, and meals. (Some drugs interact with specific fluids and timing may need to be adjusted.) If the timing of the drug is critical, stress that point. Help him to determine the best way to space drugs during the day with regard to other drug use or activities.

✦ *Special storage and preparation instructions.* Some drugs require special handling — the patient may need to wear protective gloves while applying topical products; he may need to store some drugs in the refrigerator; and he may need to cut some drugs in half, but not others. Teach the patient how to store and prepare his drugs.

✦ *Specific OTC drugs or herbal therapies to avoid.* The patient may not consider OTC drugs or herbal or alternative therapies to be actual drugs and may inadvertently take them with his prescribed medications, causing unwanted or even dangerous drug-drug interactions. To prevent these situations, explain which alternative products to avoid and give the patient that information in writing.

✦ *Special comfort measures.* Teach the patient how to cope with anticipated adverse effects to ease anxiety and avoid noncompliance with drug therapy. Telling a patient beforehand that rifampin may turn his urine orange will spare him the anxiety of discovering this effect on his own.

✦ *Safety measures.* Instruct the patient to keep drugs out of the reach of children. Also, remind him to inform every health care provider he sees about the drugs he's taking; this can prevent drug-drug interactions, overdosing with the same drug, and misdiagnosis based on drug effects.

✦ *Specific warnings about drug discontinuation:* Some drugs with a small margin of safety and drugs with particular systemic effects can't be stopped abruptly without the risk of dangerous effects. Alert the patient taking such drugs to this problem and encourage him to call his health care provider immediately if he can't continue to take the medication for any reason (such as illness, travel, or financial constraints).

✦ *Specific points about drug toxicity:* Give the patient a list of warning signs of drug toxicity, and advise him to notify the health care provider immediately if these effects occur. He also needs to know about the importance of follow-up tests or evaluations that might lead to a change in drugs or drug dosage.

Evaluation

Evaluation is part of the continual process of patient care that leads to changes in assessment, diagnosis, and intervention. You'll continually evaluate the patient for therapeutic response, the occurrence of drug adverse effects, and the occurrence of drug-drug, drug-food, drug-alternative therapy, or drug-laboratory test interactions. You'll also evaluate the efficacy of nursing interventions and the teaching program: Is the patient safe while taking this drug? Does he understand the need to take the drug on an empty stomach? In some situations, you'll evaluate the patient simply by reapplying the beginning steps of the nursing process and analyzing for change. In some cases of drug therapy, particular therapeutic drug levels also need to be evaluated.

The right patient

The first "right" to consider before administering a drug pertains to the identity of the patient. Always make sure that the patient to whom you are going to administer a drug is actually the patient that the drug is intended for. This includes not only verifying the patient's identity, but ensuring that the patient isn't allergic to the drug; isn't using a prescription drug, an over-the-counter (OTC) drug, or an alternative therapy that could interact with the drug; and isn't pregnant (if applicable).

✦ The name game

Many reported medication errors involve a mix-up in patient identity. The only way to ensure that the patient is the right patient is to check his identification. A standard approach in the facility setting—inpatient or outpatient—is to check the identification (ID) bracelet of each patient before administering a drug as well as asking the patient to state his name.

PREVENT IT

Medication error: A nurse gave morphine for pain to a patient she believed to be Mrs. Jones in room 215, bed B. Short-

ly after giving the injection, the nurse noticed that a patient on a stretcher in the hall was very uncomfortable and asking for pain medication. By checking the ID bracelet, the nurse discovered that the patient on the stretcher was Mrs. Jones. The nurse had inadvertently given the morphine injection to Mrs. Krebs, who was supposed to be in room 215, bed A. The staff member transporting Mrs. Jones had been distracted by an emergency situation after moving bed A out of the way to allow them to maneuver the stretcher into the room. Mrs. Jones was left in the hall and Mrs. Krebs' bed was out of place in the room. The nurse knew she was looking for a patient in 215B and, because the bed had been in that location, she gave the injection.

Prevention: Before giving the medication, the nurse should have checked the patient's ID bracelet and asked the patient to state her name. Frequently, on busy units, orders may be addressed to specific rooms and beds, and actual patient names may be omitted. Sometimes, diagnoses are used instead of names— "Give this med to the gallbladder in room 12," also adding to the confusion. Before you administer medication, make sure the patient's name matches the name on the medication order.

Who is it?

In some situations, a patient may not have an ID bracelet because it was removed for a procedure, it became too tight and was cut off, or it became too loose and fell off. Before administering a drug to a patient without an ID bracelet, ask the patient to state his name. Then double-check that name with the name on the medication order. Also, check the name against identification that may be posted by the patient's bed. While checking the medication order, it would be wise to get a new ID bracelet for the patient.

Asking the patient to state his name can be ineffective at times because he may be unable to answer the question. If a nurse is unable to positively identify the patient, she should withhold the medication until positive identification can be obtained.

PREVENT IT

Medication error: A nurse was pulled to work on a busy medical unit and didn't know the patients. She had digoxin (Lanoxin) to give to Mr. Murphy in room 1412, and she noticed that the patient in bed A didn't have an ID bracelet. She said, "Mr. Murphy?" The patient answered, "Yes." The nurse took that to mean that the patient was Mr. Murphy and administered the drug. It turns out that the patient in that bed had some dementia and was rather hard of hearing. He said "yes" simply as a response to someone talking to him. He was Mr. Scripture, not the intended patient, Mr. Murphy. The nurse thought she was checking appropriately and only discovered her error when she stopped at the desk and asked the clerk to make a new ID bracelet for the patient.

Prevention: When a patient isn't appropriately "labeled" for identification, ask the patient to state his name. Don't provide the name because that can lead to confusion or misunderstanding. Patients may have been medicated or may have problems that prevent them from understanding the question and answering appropriately. If you ask the patient to state his name, and the patient isn't able to reply, don't assume you know who the patient is. Check with another staff member or visitor to determine the identity of the patient before you give a drug. Remember, when in doubt, check it out.

Double trouble

It's possible that two or more patients on the same unit have the same or similar last name. If this occurs, it's important to post warnings and cautions so that all staff members are aware of the duplication of names and the possibility of mix-ups.

PREVENT IT

Medication error: *A patient care assistant (PCA) stopped by the desk to ask the nurse if "Root" could receive anything for a headache. The nurse, who was new to the unit, looked quickly through the patient list and found that there was a standing order for ibuprofen for C. Root. She got the medication, went to the room the assistant had left, checked the patient's ID bracelet, and gave the patient the drug. Half an hour later, the PCA returned to the nurse to ask again if the patient could have something for his headache. On further investigation, the nurse discovered that there were two patients named Root on that unit—Carol Root and Charles Root. She had noted "C. Root" on the patient's ID bracelet and had given the drug. Charles Root had his headache longer than was necessary, but no other harm was done.*

Prevention:With the reality of a nursing shortage and the possibility that nurses may float to different areas and may not be familiar with a particular unit at a given time, it's very important to post warnings when patients with the same last name are on the same unit. In an ideal world, it would be against policy to have two patients with the same name on the same unit. In reality, however, duplication can occur. To prevent a dangerous mix-up, post notices on the medication orders, in the nursing Kardex, and at the nurses' station. Get into the habit of always referring to these patients by first and last names. Make sure the ID bracelets for these patients contain the first name (not just an initial) and last name. Alert the pharmacy to ensure that it clearly identifies the name of the patient—by first and last name—and marks the drugs clearly.

With special populations of patients, verifying identity can be more difficult. Children, older patients, and long-term patients commonly are referred to by their first names. It's much more likely that a unit may have several patients with the same first name than with the same last name.

PREVENT IT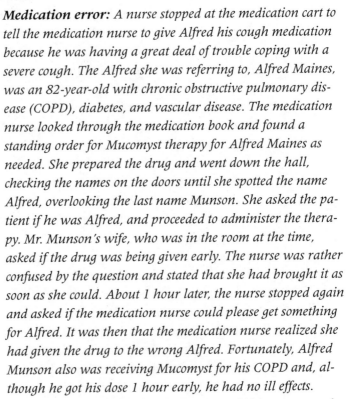

Medication error: A nurse stopped at the medication cart to tell the medication nurse to give Alfred his cough medication because he was having a great deal of trouble coping with a severe cough. The Alfred she was referring to, Alfred Maines, was an 82-year-old with chronic obstructive pulmonary disease (COPD), diabetes, and vascular disease. The medication nurse looked through the medication book and found a standing order for Mucomyst therapy for Alfred Maines as needed. She prepared the drug and went down the hall, checking the names on the doors until she spotted the name Alfred, overlooking the last name Munson. She asked the patient if he was Alfred, and proceeded to administer the therapy. Mr. Munson's wife, who was in the room at the time, asked if the drug was being given early. The nurse was rather confused by the question and stated that she had brought it as soon as she could. About 1 hour later, the nurse stopped again and asked if the medication nurse could please get something for Alfred. It was then that the medication nurse realized she had given the drug to the wrong Alfred. Fortunately, Alfred Munson also was receiving Mucomyst for his COPD and, although he got his dose 1 hour early, he had no ill effects.

Prevention: The medication nurse could have prevented the error if she had verified the patient's full name, checked his ID bracelet for verification, and checked the medication record to make sure the drug hadn't been given already. The nurse requesting the drug could have prevented the error by clearly stating the full name of the patient who needed the drug. Always check the patient's ID bracelet and make sure that the information matches the order and the drug you are about to administer.

Encore patients

Identification errors aren't limited to inpatient settings. Many procedures are now performed on outpatients, including surgeries, diagnostic procedures, and chemotherapeutic regimens. In many settings, patients receive an ID bracelet as the first step in the admission process before a procedure. In other areas, when patients come frequently for repeated procedures, such as hemodialysis or chemotherapy, this practice may be omitted. In these settings, it's important to check for some form of identification before giving medications.

PREVENT IT

Medication error: John Grice came to the Cancer Outpatient Clinic for the sixth in a series of antineoplastic treatments. The clinic was crowded with patients and their significant others. A smiling nurse approached John, started his I.V. line, and gave him a full dose of mitomycin I.V., chatting with him while the drug infused and asking about problems that may have come up after the last treatment. John was resting in a reclining chair when his wife heard another nurse calling for John Grice. She went to the nurse, who was looking for this patient, and told her that Mr. Grice had already received his injection. The patient and his wife had recognized the nurse who administered the drug on previous visits. It turned out that the nurse who administered the drug recognized John from previous visits also, but she thought his name was John Stahl and had given him the drug intended for that patient. The patients in this clinic aren't given ID bracelets for each visit; the nurse assumed she remembered the patient correctly, and the patient assumed that the nurse knew who he was. I.V. fluids were administered rapidly, and Mr. Grice was monitored closely for several hours to assess for any complications caused by the wrong medication being given.

Prevention: No nurse can remember the names of all the patients she sees over several weeks. This nurse, on a very busy day, was convinced that she knew the patient, and the patient, who responded to "John," seemed to know her, so she proceeded without checking further. Several outpatient facilities in which regular procedures are performed don't use ID bracelets for identification. Many times patients don't bring their driver's licenses or other identification with them. The clinic in this situation learned from this mistake and developed a plan to prevent such errors in the future. It gave patients ID cards when they checked in with the secretary; the nurses would then check the ID cards against the medication orders before administering drugs. So far, this strategy is working.

Pharmacy errors

Errors in identification have also been reported in outpatient pharmacies. Because they're in such short supply, pharmacists are often overworked and under a great deal of pressure. Sometimes, some of the checks that once effectively prevented problems may not be followed as faithfully. It's important to check the drugs that patients are taking at home to make sure that the drugs they received are the drugs that were prescribed.

PREVENT IT

Medication error: Sarah Gilbert dropped off her prescriptions at the drugstore to be refilled while she was shopping in the mall. Her health care provider had re-ordered 100 mcg levothyroxine (Synthroid), 20 mg fluoxetine (Prozac), and 0.625 mg conjugated estrogen (Premarin), all of which she had been taking for some time. He told her that some of these drugs were now available in a generic form and that they might not look like those she was used to taking. When she picked up the drugs, she asked for "Gilbert," and was given a bag with directions stapled to it. She paid for the prescriptions and went home. Because she had been taking these drugs for quite some time, she threw away the printed instructions. The drugs in the bag did look quite different from her usual pills, but she assumed this was because they were generic. She didn't read the labels because she didn't have her glasses on and she knew how to take the drugs anyway. Two weeks later, she didn't feel right and called her health care provider, who asked her to come in and bring the medications she was taking. Not only were the drugs that she had taken intended for Jason Gilbert, she hadn't been taking her usual medications for the past 2 weeks. Instead, she was taking clonazepam (Klonopin), hydrochlorothiazide (HydroDIURIL), and nifedipine (Procardia). These medications were stopped, she was evaluated, and she restarted her regular medications.

Prevention: Patients picking up prescriptions should be asked for identification, whether it's an insurance card, a driver's license, or another ID. Pharmacies can be busy and hectic, and it's easy to see how name mix-ups can occur. If a patient reports new signs or symptoms or a return of old problems after getting prescriptions filled, it's a good idea to ask to see the medications. All patients should be encouraged to bring their medications with them when they see their health care providers, and these drugs should be checked against the record.

✦ History issues

Medication errors can occur when elements of the patient's history have been omitted, missed, or overlooked. These elements can be important in determining if a patient is the right candidate for the drug that's being ordered. The elements that should be assessed before giving a medication include allergies (all types) and the nature of the reactions, use of other drugs (prescription, OTC, illicit, and herbal), the patient's age and weight, and pregnancy status (if applicable).

Allergies

A drug allergy occurs when the body develops antibodies to a particular drug, causing an immune response when the body is re-exposed to that drug. Drug allergies generally fall into four categories:

✦ *anaphylactic reactions,* which can involve hives, increased heart rate, increased blood pressure, dilated pupils, difficulty breathing, and respiratory arrest

✦ *cytotoxic reactions,* which can involve liver or renal dysfunction or damage to blood-forming cells in bone marrow

✦ *serum-sickness reactions,* which involve rash, fever, swollen and painful joints, and edema

✦ *delayed allergic reactions,* which can involve rash, hives, and swollen joints occurring several hours after exposure.

An allergic reaction can range from discomfort to death. Patients with respiratory or cardiovascular diseases or renal or liver dysfunction are at significant risk if an allergic reaction occurs. If possible, patients should be protected from exposure not only to the specific drug that caused an allergic reaction, but also to other drugs in that pharmacologic class. For exam-

ple, if a patient suffered an allergic reaction to penicillin, he shouldn't receive ampicillin either.

A patient can't have a drug allergy to a drug that he
has never taken. The body has to develop antibodies to
a drug after it has been exposed to it. When listing a
patient's allergies, it's important to find out when the
drug allergy developed: Was it after a long-term use of
the drug? Was it after the second exposure to the
drug?

PREVENT IT

Medication error: A college student was seen in the University Health Service with a severe sore throat that cultured positive for streptococcus, which is sensitive to penicillin. The
nurse practitioner called in an order for penicillin; however,
the student called back to report that he was allergic to penicillin. While talking to the student about the allergy, the
nurse learned that the student had never taken penicillin but,
because most of his relatives were allergic to the drug, he assumed that he was as well. The patient was given the penicillin and a list of adverse effects — hives, increased fever, and
difficulty breathing — to report immediately if they occurred.

Prevention: The student responded well to the penicillin
and recovered quickly with no adverse effects. The student
could have been started on the drug sooner if the nature of his
"allergy" had been understood. The next time the student is
given penicillin, the health care provider may want to monitor him closely because that would be the time that a reaction
might occur.

Reaction versus response

The patient may report that he has a drug allergy
when what he's actually experiencing is the effects of
the drug. When taking a history, it's important to ask

the patient not only when he had an allergic reaction to the drug, but also what the reaction actually was.

PREVENT IT

Medication error: Mrs. Olsen told the nurse who was about to administer furosemide (Lasix) for her heart failure that she had taken that drug before and was allergic to it. The nurse checked the patient record and didn't find mention of this allergy in the chart. The patient, in response to questioning, reported that she forgot about the allergy until the nurse told her that she was giving her Lasix. The nurse put in a call to the prescribing health care provider to get a different order to help resolve this patient's edema and help her heart failure. The health care provider was attending a seminar and didn't call back for several hours. Meanwhile, Mrs. Olsen developed mild respiratory distress. When reached, the health care provider remembered prescribing Lasix in the past for this patient with success and was quite surprised to learn about the allergy. Upon further questioning, the nurse discovered that the "allergy" that Mrs. Olsen was reporting was that the drug made her go to the bathroom frequently. The patient thought that the increased urination was an allergic reaction and not the drug's desired effect. With this clarified, the patient received Lasix.

Prevention: When the patient reported an allergy to the drug, the nurse should have asked what that allergic reaction was. Was the response actually an allergy, or was it a desired or adverse effect of the drug? This patient could have started treatment earlier if the nature of the allergic response had been clarified.

Allergy alert systems

Health care facilities have safeguards in place to alert health care personnel about patient allergies — allergy alert stickers and labels that are processed when a patient comes under the care of that facility. The patient chart allergy warning usually lists drugs that shouldn't be given to the patient. A brightly colored sticker may be placed on the medication record, in the Kardex, or on the patient's door or bed, or a special ID bracelet may be used to alert personnel that this patient has allergies.

In large facilities, where many care providers may interact with the patient, these warning stickers can be a mixed blessing. Health care providers can come to rely on these alerts and labels instead of relying on the patient or their own judgment. It's important when administering a drug to ask the patient directly if he has allergies. Relying on the efficiency and accuracy of the system isn't an error-proof way of noting allergies.

PREVENT IT

Medication error: Bob Frye was admitted to a large teaching hospital's medical unit with severe cellulitis. The admitting physician sent an admission workup with the patient, which the unit secretary put in the patient's chart. The admitting nurse did the patient workup and wrote her admission note. The patient was allergic to penicillins and cephalosporins. The initial allergic reaction to penicillin had been a life-threatening anaphylactic response. Although the nurse noted this in the chart, she was busy with four admissions that afternoon and relied on the unit secretary to put allergy alerts on the chart and the medication sheet and place a special wristband on the patient, which the facility used to identify allergies. The secretary, who was also very busy with admissions and discharges, didn't have time to place all the notifications and left a note for the evening secretary to complete several tasks. A medical student was also assigned to admit Mr. Frye and did his medical workup, but forgot to ask about allergies. Noticing that the patient had an admitting physician and nurse workup in the chart and no allergy alerts had *been posted, the medical student wrote "NKA" — no known allergies — on his history form. The resident, who followed the student and knew the student was quite thorough, also wrote NKA, based on the student's history form. An infectious disease fellow also saw Mr. Frye, who was tired of answering questions and being examined. They also saw the student's NKA and noted no allergies in their workup. Cephalosporin was ordered for the patient. The medication nurse who went to give the drug had to wake Mr. Frye and didn't question him. Later, she stated that there were no allergy alerts on the chart, nursing Kardex, medication sheet, or patient ID bracelet and she had felt safe giving the drug. Mr. Frye broke out in hives and developed a high fever. It was then discovered that he had a cephalosporin allergy that hadn't been relayed properly. He was treated with diphenhydramine and the cephalosporin was stopped.*

Prevention: Relying on computers, warning labels, and red flags becomes too easy. Units are very busy and many nurses are overworked and under strain. These conveniences are designed to save time and prevent problems. It's important to remember, however, that they all rely on human input, and all humans can make mistakes. The absence of a warning label, red flag, or special wristband doesn't mean that the patient has no allergies. Always ask the patient if he has allergies before giving a medication. This is especially important with penicillins, cephalosporins, narcotics, and nonsteroidal anti-inflammatory drugs, which are the most reported allergy-causing drugs. If the patient can't respond or is unreliable, check old records and ask family members or caregivers. Satisfy yourself that the information you have is accurate.

Updating information

Patients are dynamic, as stated earlier. Their responses, environment, and status may be constantly fluctuating. It's important to remember that their allergy status can also fluctuate; as they're exposed to more drugs, their body's response to drugs can also change. Don't rely on old records or histories to get the information that you need to know before giving a drug. Ask the patient if he has known drug allergies every time you give a drug.

PREVENT IT

Medication error: Carl Thomas was readmitted to the rehabilitation unit for the third time. The staff recognized the name and the diagnosis: postmotorcycle accident paralysis. To save time, the staff retrieved his old medical records and prepared his chart before he arrived on the unit. An allergy ID bracelet had been prepared, the warnings were posted on the chart and bed per facility policy, and the nursing Kardex was marked. On the second day of his admission, the patient complained of a bad headache and the nurse noted that a standing order for aspirin had been written on admission. She gave the patient the aspirin and, within 2 hours, he had developed a rash and fever and was complaining of difficulty breathing. The staff began supportive measures, including blood cultures to determine if an infection was the cause of the problem. When Carl was more comfortable, he asked what he had been given for his headache. He then reported that he was allergic to aspirin. Although the chart was carefully reviewed, there was no notation of this allergy. Carl reported that he hadn't been allergic to this drug before, but had developed this allergy about 3 months ago, and his physician informed him that he couldn't take aspirin again. Because the staff knew the patient and felt comfortable with him on admission, some of the patient history questions that are normally asked were omitted because they thought that this information had already been recorded.

Prevention: Always ask a patient if he has known allergies to medications before giving a drug. Don't rely on old *records, warning signs, or special wristbands. This patient had all of those warnings, but they weren't up-to-date. In the long run, the nurse administering a drug is the one responsible for ensuring that the patient is the right patient—which also means a patient who isn't allergic to the drug that's being administered.*

Using drugs together

Many drugs are known to interfere with other drugs. This can occur when one drug blocks or enhances the absorption, metabolism, or excretion of another drug. It can also occur when a drug has an effect that enhances or opposes the effect of another drug. There are many sources of drugs other than prescription, and the nurse needs to be aware of all drug use by patients to whom she'll administer medications so she can assess the situation for potential drug interactions.

The most common errors involving such drug interactions occur when a patient is given a drug that interacts with an OTC drug, an herbal therapy, or a routine medication that the patient neglected to report. Although it's difficult or impossible to question the patient about all medication use each time a drug is given in the hospital setting, it's very important to find out that information and record it in the patient's chart when the patient first comes into the facility.

In the outpatient setting, the drug history should be reviewed each time the patient is seen. Specific questions should be developed to ascertain the use of other drugs. Simply asking the patient if he's taking other medications or drugs may not give the information that's needed and could affect the patient's progress and therapy.

Problems with OTC drugs

The Food and Drug Administration approves a drug for over-the-counter (OTC) use when it's found to be "safe when used as directed." Problems can arise when:

✦ directions aren't read or followed properly
✦ the drug masks the signs and symptoms that are needed to properly signal a problem
✦ patients don't consider these products as drugs, and neglect to mention them when asked if they're using drugs or medications.

Over-the-counter drugs

The availability of OTC drugs is staggering. Patients are able to self-diagnose and self-treat many common complaints ranging from headache to constipation, gastric upset, allergies, and fungal infections. OTC drugs are widely advertised, and most people see them as commonplace. (See *Problems with OTC drugs*.)

When obtaining a drug history, you should always ask specifically if the patient is using OTC medications. You may even need to give a few examples, such as Tylenol, Aleve, ExLax, Dimetapp, or Pepcid, to stir the patient's memory. (See *Precautions for OTC drugs, pages 60 to 64*.)

PREVENT IT

Medication error: Jim Hermann had been stabilized on acebutolol (Sectral) to manage his hypertension for more than 6 months. He came to the clinic for a routine blood pressure

(Text continues on page 64.)

✦

Precautions for OTC drugs

Using over-the-counter (OTC) drugs can cause drug-drug interactions. When taking a drug history, be sure to ask about the patient's use of OTC drugs. The chart below lists ingredients in some OTC drugs, the drugs they may react with, and the possible reactions.

OTC INGREDIENT	REACTING DRUGS	POSSIBLE REACTION
acetaminophen	Oral anticoagulants	Increased bleeding
	Barbiturates, carbamazepine, hydantoins, rifampin, sulfinpyrazone	Hepatoxicity, decreased therapeutic effects
	Zidovudine	Decreased effectiveness
aluminum hydroxide	Other oral drugs	Decreased absorption and effectiveness
	Corticosteroids, diflunisal, digoxin, iron, isoniazid, penicillamine, phenothiazines, ranitidine, tetracyclines	Decreased therapeutic effects of these drugs
	Benzodiazepines	Increased effects and risk of toxicity
aspirin	Oral anticoagulants, heparin	Increased bleeding
	Corticosteroids, phenylbutazone, alcohol, nonsteroidal anti-inflammatory drugs	Increased risk of GI ulceration
	Carbonic anhydrase inhibitors, furosemide	Risk of salicylate toxicity

Precautions for OTC drugs *(continued)*

OTC INGREDIENT	REACTING DRUGS	POSSIBLE REACTION
aspirin *(continued)*	Corticosteroids, acetazolamide, methazolamide, antacids	Decreased aspirin levels and effects
	Methotrexate	Increased toxicity when combined with aspirin
	Valproic acid	Increased effects
	Sulfonylureas, insulin	Increased glucose lowering effects
	Beta-adrenergic blockers	Decreased antihypertensive effects
	Probenecid, sulfinpyrazone	Decreased uricosuric effect
	Spironolactone, furosemide	Decreased diuretic effect
	Nitroglycerin	Possible hypotension
caffeine	Cimetidine, oral contraceptives, disulfiram, ciprofloxacin, mexiletine	Increased caffeine, central nervous system (CNS) effects
	Theophylline, clozapine	Increased serum levels and risk of toxicity from these drugs
cascara	Other laxatives	Severe diarrhea, malabsorption syndromes
castor oil	Other laxatives	Severe diarrhea, malabsorption syndromes

(continued)

Precautions for OTC drugs *(continued)*

OTC INGREDIENT	REACTING DRUGS	POSSIBLE REACTION
chlorpheniramine	CNS depressants, alcohol	Increased CNS depression, dizziness, drowsiness
dextromethorphan	Monoamine oxidase (MAO) inhibitors	Hypotension, hyperpyrexia, nausea, myoclonic leg jerks, coma
diphenhydramine	MAO inhibitors	Increased anticholinergic effects
docusate	Other laxatives	Severe diarrhea, malabsorption syndromes
ibuprofen	Lithium	Increased toxic effects of lithium
	Furosemide, bumetanide, ethacrynic acid	Decreased diuretic effects
	Beta-adrenergic blockers	Decreased antihypertensive effects
	Digoxin	Possible increased digoxin levels
	Anticoagulants	Possible increased bleeding
ketoprofen	Lithium	Increased toxic effects of lithium
	Furosemide, bumetanide, ethacrynic acid	Decreased diuretic effects
	Beta-adrenergic blockers	Decreased antihypertensive effects

Precautions for OTC drugs *(continued)*

OTC INGREDIENT	REACTING DRUGS	POSSIBLE REACTION
ketoprofen *(continued)*	Digoxin	Possible increased digoxin levels
	Anticoagulants	Possible increased bleeding
magnesium hydroxide	Other oral drugs	Decreased absorption and effectiveness
	Corticosteroids, digoxin, iron, penicillamine, nitrofurantoin, tetracyclines	Decreased therapeutic effects of these drugs
mineral oil	Docusate	Increased risk of mineral oil absorption
	Fat-soluble vitamins	Decreased absorption of these vitamins
naproxen	Lithium	Increased toxic effects of lithium
	Furosemide, bumetanide, ethacrynic acid	Decreased diuretic effects
	Beta-adrenergic blockers	Decreased antihypertensive effects
	Digoxin	Possible increased digoxin levels
	Anticoagulants	Possible increased bleeding

(continued)

Precautions for OTC drugs *(continued)*

OTC INGREDIENT	REACTING DRUGS	POSSIBLE REACTION
pseudoephedrine	MAO inhibitors, guanethidine, furazoladine	Increased hypertension
	Methyldopa	Decreased antihypertensive effect
	Urine alkalinizers	Increased effects of pseudoephedrine
	Urine acidifiers	Decreased effects of pseudoephedrine
psyllium	Other laxatives	Severe diarrhea, malabsorption syndromes
senna	Other laxatives	Severe diarrhea, malabsorption syndromes

check, and his blood pressure was found to be elevated at 160/94 mm Hg, markedly higher than that over the past 6 months. When asked, Jim denied the use of other medications. After much discussion, it was decided to add a diuretic to his medication regimen and have him return in 2 weeks for another check. He called the health care provider 10 days later to report that he was very weak and light-headed and felt awful. When he arrived at the clinic, his blood pressure was 110/68 mm Hg — below his normal baseline. The nurse couldn't figure out how a mild diuretic could lower his pressure so much. She asked if anything else had changed, and he reported that his cold was gone. He had been self-treating a cold with Actifed Allergy. This combination product contains pseudoephedrine and diphenhydramine, both of which can affect blood pressure. He hadn't reported the use of the drug because he said he didn't think of it as a drug; he was thinking only of things that the doctor had prescribed. The ingredients in this drug had counteracted his blood pressure medication, accounting for the increased blood pressure on his first visit. Hence, he had been given an additional blood pressure-lowering drug, which was too strong after he stopped taking the Actifed Allergy.

Prevention: Jim Hermann's beliefs about OTC drugs are very common. Although asked if he was taking other medications, he should have been asked specifically if he was taking OTC medications such as cold remedies. If health care providers are unaware that patients are using OTC drugs, they may give the patients other drugs to counter the effect of the OTC products, believing that the effects suggest a physical disorder. Prescription drugs may be stopped or the dosages altered because the effects of the drug aren't the expected outcome, when the actual problem is a drug interaction with an OTC drug. These complications can be costly in terms of the patient's health and finances. When a patient is prescribed a medication, it may be helpful to provide a patient-teaching guide to inform him about the prescribed drug as well as potential interactions with OTC and other drugs. (See Sample patient-teaching aid, *pages 66 and 67.)*

Herbal therapy

There's a growing movement toward the use of "natural" substances to treat diseases. Television and radio ads, magazine spreads, and talk shows focus on the use of many herbal therapies to treat hypertension, menopause, depression, high cholesterol, and other medical problems. Consumers are urged to take control of their own health and use these products to self-treat many ailments and to avoid the use of "drugs" and other medical procedures.

Sample patient-teaching aid

Incorporating critical information about potential drug interactions with over-the-counter (OTC) drugs or herbal therapies into patient-teaching materials can prevent medication errors from occurring. Here's a sample teaching aid.

Patient name: Janice Hermann

You should know the following information about the drug that has been prescribed for you.

Drug name: acebutolol

This drug is being given to help lower your blood pressure. It's called a beta-adrenergic blocker.

How to pronounce this name: ah se byoo' toe loll

Other names that this drug is known by: Sectral

Instructions to follow for your safety:

✦ Take this drug two times a day with meals. If you miss a dose, make it up as soon as you remember. If you miss doses for an entire day, don't make up the doses. Don't take more than two tablets each day.

✦ Don't stop taking this medication without talking to your health care provider. Serious effects could occur if you suddenly stop taking this drug. If your health care provider wants you to discontinue this drug, your doses will be tapered gradually over about 2 weeks.

✦ You may experience the following side effects: dizziness or weakness (if these occur, avoid driving or performing dangerous activities); loss of appetite or upset stomach (taking the drug with meals should help); nightmares, depression, sexual dysfunction (talk to your health care provider if these become a problem).

✦ Report to your health care provider: difficulty breathing, night cough, swelling of extremities, slow pulse, confusion, rash, fever, or sore throat.

✦ Don't use OTC drugs called nonsteroidal anti-inflammatory agents— these include such products as aspirin, *Motrin, Advil,* and *Aleve.* These drugs could increase the blood pressure-lowering effect of your pre-scribed medication and cause serious problems. If you feel that you need one of these drugs, talk to your health care provider for one that would be appropriate.

✦ Don't use oral contraceptives (birth control pills) while taking this drug; serious adverse effects could occur. Instead, use barrier protection.

Sample patient-teaching aid *(continued)*

✦ Tell every health care provider who's taking care of you that you're using this drug. Also, tell every provider about your use of OTC drugs or herbal therapies so that potential negative side effects can be avoided.
✦ Keep this drug, and all medications, out of the reach of children.

Although many traditional drugs used today are also naturally occurring chemicals, the Food and Drug Administration (FDA) has tested and evaluated them for efficacy and safety. The FDA doesn't treat herbal products as drugs and doesn't subject them to the testing and quality control procedures that are required of more traditional medications. Although the advertising of these products isn't as tightly regulated as that for traditional drugs, all advertisements must contain a disclaimer: "These products have not been tested by the FDA." Many of these products have been used for hundreds of years as home remedies for various conditions. Some products contain chemicals that have been developed into prescription drugs, and others contain chemicals that haven't yet been tested for efficacy and safety. In many cases, there's no scientific evidence of the safety or effectiveness of these products.

There have been increasing reports of drug interactions between herbal products and other drugs. The FDA reports these problems and is being urged by many consumer safety groups to adopt a more active role in controlling herbal products. (See *Precautions for herbal therapy,* pages 68 to 89.)

In some situations, a patient may use herbal products for a condition that's already being treated by oth-

(Text continues on page 88.)

Precautions for herbal therapy

For some herbal substances, specific interactions with conventional drugs have been reported. Checking for the possibility of such interactions may help to prevent medication errors and may explain unexpected adverse effects or lack of

HERBAL SUBSTANCE	REPORTED USES
alfalfa	*Topical:* healing ointment, relieving arthritis pain *Oral:* treating arthritis, gaining strength
allspice	*Topical:* anesthetic for teeth and gums; soothing sore joints and muscles *Oral:* treating indigestion, flatulence, diarrhea, fatigue Seizures have been reported with excessive dosage.
aloe leaves	*Topical:* treating burns, healing wounds *Oral:* treating chronic constipation
anise	*Oral:* relieving dry cough, treating flatulence
apple	*Oral:* controlling blood glucose, treating constipation
arnica gel	*Topical:* relieving pain from muscle and soft-tissue injury
ashwagandha	*Oral:* enhancing mental and physical function, general tonic; used to protect cells during cancer chemotherapy and radiation therapy Contraindicated in pregnant and breast-feeding women
astragalus	*Oral:* increasing stamina and energy; improving immune function and resistance to disease Don't use with fever, acute infection, live vaccinations.

anticipated therapeutic effects in the patient. The following chart lists herbs and their reported uses and interactions.

REPORTED INTERACTIONS

Monitor patients on antiepileptic drugs.

Monitor patients closely if used with antidiabetic drugs.

(continued)

Precautions for herbal therapy *(continued)*

HERBAL SUBSTANCE	REPORTED USES
barberry	*Oral:* antidiarrheal, antipyretic, cough suppressant Risk of spontaneous abortion if taken during pregnancy
bayberry	*Topical:* promoting wound healing *Oral:* stimulant, emetic antidiarrheal
bee pollen	*Oral:* enhancing athletic performance
bilberry	*Oral:* treating diabetes, cardiovascular disorders, diabetic retinopathy, cataracts, and night blindness; lowering cholesterol and triglycerides
birch bark	*Topical:* treating infected wounds, cuts *Oral:* as tea for relieving stomach ache
blackberry	*Oral:* as tea for generalized healing, treating diabetes
black cohosh	*Oral:* relieving symptoms of menopause, premenstrual syndrome (PMS) Contains alcohol, which can cause dizziness and vision disturbances; don't use in pregnant or breast-feeding women.
borage	*Oral:* relieving symptoms of menopause Associated with seizures, liver dysfunction.
bromelain	*Oral:* treating inflammation, sports injuries; upper respiratory infections, premenstrual syndrome, adjunct to cancer therapy
burdock	*Oral:* treating diabetes, atropine-like effects; uterine stimulant
camomile	*Topical:* treating wounds, ulcers, conjunctivitis *Oral:* treating migraines and gastric cramps, relieving anxiety .

REPORTED INTERACTIONS

Monitor patients with known allergies; severe allergic reactions are common.

Monitor patients for effects if taken with antidiabetic or cholesterol-lowering drugs.

Monitor patients closely if on antidiabetic drugs.

Don't combine with disulfiram or metrondiazole; don't use with hormone replacement therapy (HRT) or oral contraceptives.

Don't use with antiepileptic drugs and drugs that can cause liver impairment.

Don't use with HRT or oral contraceptives; use caution with nonsteroidal anti-inflammatory drugs (NSAIDs).

Monitor patients closely if taking antidiabetic drugs or anticholinergics.

Monitor patients on anticoagulants; this herb contains coumarin. Monitor patients on antidepressants; herb known to cause depression.

(continued)

Precautions for herbal therapy *(continued)*

HERBAL SUBSTANCE	REPORTED USES
capsicum	*Topical:* external analgesic *Oral:* treating bowel disorders, chronic laryngitis, peripheral vascular disease
catnip leaves	*Oral:* treating bronchitis, diarrhea
cat's claw	*Oral:* treating allergies, arthritis; adjunct treatment in cancer, acquired immunodeficiency syndrome (AIDS). Don't use in pregnant or breast-feeding women and in patients receiving transplants.
cayenne pepper	*Topical:* treating burns, wounds; relieving toothache pain
celery	*Oral:* lowering blood glucose, acts as a diuretic, may lower potassium levels
chaste tree berry	*Oral:* progesterone-like effects; treating PMS, symptoms of menopause; may stimulate lactation
chicken soup	*Oral:* breaking up respiratory secretions, bronchodilator, relieving anxiety
chicory	*Oral:* treating digestive tract problems, gout; stimulates bile secretions
Chinese angelica	*Oral:* general tonic; treating anemia, PMS, symptoms of menopause; also used as an antihypertensive and laxative
chondroitin	*Oral:* treating osteoarthritis and related disorders
chong cao fungi	*Oral:* antioxidant, promoting stamina and sexual function Don't use in children.

REPORTED INTERACTIONS

Monitor for bleeding with oral anticoagulants.

Monitor patients closely if on antidiabetic drugs or diuretics.

Use caution with HRT and oral contraceptives; don't combine with beta blockers or antihypertensives.

Monitor patients on antihypertensives or vasodilators for toxic effects; use caution with HRT and oral contraceptives.

Monitor patients on anticoagulants because of the risk of increased bleeding.

(continued)

Precautions for herbal therapy *(continued)*

HERBAL SUBSTANCE	REPORTED USES
coleus forskohlii	*Oral:* treating asthma, hypertension, eczema Don't use in patients with hypotension or peptic ulcers.
comfrey	*Topical:* treating wounds, cuts, ulcers *Oral:* gargle for tonsillitis
coriander	*Oral:* losing weight, lowering blood glucose
creatine	*Oral:* general tonic for increasing stamina and energy, increasing athletic performance Push fluids to prevent renal dysfunction.
damiana	*Oral:* increasing muscle strength; aphrodisiac in males; increasing energy Don't use in children.
dandelion root	*Oral:* treating liver and kidney problems; decreasing lactation (after delivery or with weaning); lowering blood glucose
devil's claw	*Oral:* relieving symptoms of menopause, PMS; increases stomach acid levels
dehydroepiandrosterone	*Oral:* slowing aging, improving vigor, androgenic effects
Di huang	*Oral:* treating diabetes mellitus
dong quai	*Oral:* relieving symptoms of menopause, PMS
dried root bark of lycium Chinese mill	*Oral:* lowering blood glucose and blood cholesterol
echinacea	*Oral:* treating colds, flu; stimulating or suppressing the immune system Avoid use in patients with tuberculosis, AIDS, and systemic lupus erythematosus.

REPORTED INTERACTIONS

Use caution with antihistamines or antihypertensives; severe reactions have been reported.

Associated with bladder cancer and tumors; herb shouldn't be ingested.

Monitor patients also using antidiabetic drugs.

Known to interact with actions of NSAIDs, cimetidine, probenecid, trimethroprim, and other nephrotoxic drugs.

Interferes with vitamin B_{12} absorption.

Monitor patients on antidiabetic drugs.

Increased stomach acid can interfere with absorption of many drugs; monitor patients closely for drug effectiveness; don't use with HRT or oral contraceptives.

Monitor patients also on androgens for possible toxic effects.

Monitor patients on antidiabetic drugs.

Don't use with oral anticoagulants; severe bleeding may occur.

Monitor patients on antidiabetic or cholesterol-lowering drugs.

Don't use with hepatotoxic drugs; severe liver toxicity can occur. Don't use with antifungals or immunosuppressants.

(continued)

Precautions for herbal therapy *(continued)*

HERBAL SUBSTANCE	REPORTED USES
elder bark or flowers	*Topical:* gargle for tonsillitis, pharyngitis *Oral:* treating fever, chills
ephedra	*Oral:* increasing energy, relieving fatigue Associated with severe complications; withdrawn in many states.
ergot	*Oral:* treating migraine headaches, menstrual problems, hemorrhage
eucalyptus	*Topical:* treating wounds *Oral:* decreasing respiratory secretions, suppressing cough
evening primrose	*Oral:* treating PMS, menopause, rheumatoid arthritis, diabetic neuropathy
false unicorn root	*Oral:* relieving symptoms of menopause, PMS
fennel	*Oral:* treating colic, gout, flatulence; enhancing lactation
fenugreek	*Oral:* lowering blood cholesterol, reducing blood glucose, aiding in healing
feverfew	*Oral:* treating arthritis, fever, migraine Don't use immediately before or after surgery because of risk of bleeding.
fish oil	*Oral:* treating coronary diseases, arthritis, colitis, depression, attention deficit hyperactivity disorder
gamboge	*Oral:* suppressing appetite, lowering cholesterol
garlic	*Oral:* treating colds, diuretic; preventing coronary artery disease, intestinal antiseptic, anticoagulant

REPORTED INTERACTIONS

Use caution with NSAIDs.

Avoid use with antihypertensive drugs, beta blockers, anticholinergics, thyroid medications, and antidiabetic drugs.

Monitor patients on HRT, oral contraceptives, triptans for migraine relief, or oral anticoagulants.

Don't use with phenothiazines or antidepressants because of the increased risk of seizure. Monitor patients on HRT.

Don't combine with estrogens or progestins (HRT, oral contraceptive, replacement therapy); may alter uterine effects.

Monitor patients on antidiabetic or cholesterol-lowering drugs.

Don't use with oral anticoagulants because of the risk of increased bleeding.

Monitor patients on cholesterol-lowering drugs.

Monitor patients on antidiabetic drugs or oral anticoagulants for toxic effects.

(continued)

Precautions for herbal therapy *(continued)*

HERBAL SUBSTANCE	REPORTED USES
ginger	*Oral:* treating nausea, motion sickness May increase risk of miscarriage
ginkgo	*Oral:* vascular dilator, improving blood flow to the brain and cognitive functioning, treating and preventing Alzheimer's disease
ginkobe	*Oral:* improving concentration and memory
ginseng	*Oral:* aphrodisiac, mood elevator, tonic; antihypertensive; decreasing cholesterol levels
glucosamine	*Oral:* treating osteoarthritis and joint diseases, usually with chondroitin
goldenrod leaves	*Oral:* treating renal disease, rheumatism, sore throat, eczema
goldenseal	*Oral:* lowering blood glucose, aiding healing, treating colds, flu, cystitis High doses have caused paralysis.
gotu kola	*Topical:* treating cellulitis, wounds, pressure ulcers
grape seed extract	*Oral:* treating allergies, asthma, improving circulation
green leaf tea	*Oral:* antioxidant; preventing cancer and coronary disease
guayusa	*Oral:* lowering blood glucose, losing weight

REPORTED INTERACTIONS

Don't give with anticoagulants because of the risk of increased bleeding.

Don't give with aspirin, NSAIDs, or oral anticoagulants because of the increased risk of bleeding. Serious reactions are possible with phenytoin, carbamazepine, phenobarbital, tricyclic antidepressants, and monoamine oxidase (MAO) inhibitors.

Don't use with aspirin, NSAIDs, or anticoagulants because of the increased risk of bleeding. Risk of headaches and manic attacks with phenelzine and MAO inhibitors. Additive and toxic effects with estrogens and corticosteroids. Decreased effectiveness of digoxin. Increased irritability with caffeine or caffeine-containing products.

Don't use with anticoagulants because of the risk of increased bleeding.

Don't use with anticoagulants because of the risk of increased bleeding.

Don't use with anticoagulants because of the risk of increased bleeding.

Monitor patients on antidiabetic drugs.

(continued)

Precautions for herbal therapy *(continued)*

HERBAL SUBSTANCE	REPORTED USES
hawthorn	*Oral:* treating angina, blood pressure, arrhythmias; lowering cholesterol levels
hops	*Oral:* sedative, aiding healing, altering blood glucose
horehound	*Oral:* expectorant; treating respiratory problems, GI disorders
horse chestnut seed	*Oral:* treating varicose veins, hemorrhoids
hyssop	*Topical:* treating cold sores, genital herpes, burns, wounds *Oral:* treating coughs, colds, indigestion, flatulence
Java plum	*Oral:* treating diabetes mellitus
jojoba	*Topical:* promoting hair growth, relieving skin problems Toxic if ingested.
juniper berries	*Oral:* increasing appetite, aiding digestion, diuretic, urinary tract disinfectant, lowering blood glucose
kava	*Oral:* treating anxiety, stress, restlessness Don't use with Parkinson's disease or history of stroke.
kudzu	*Oral:* decreasing the craving for alcohol
lavender	*Topical:* astringent for minor cuts, burns *Oral:* treating insomnia, restlessness
licorice	*Oral:* preventing thirst, soothing coughs, treating chronic fatigue syndrome, duodenal ulcer Don't use for renal or liver disease, hypertension, or coronary artery disease and in pregnant or breast-feeding patients.

REPORTED INTERACTIONS

Use caution with digoxin or angiotensin-converting enzyme inhibitors; may enhance effects. Monitor patients on cholesterol-lowering drugs.

Monitor patients on antidiabetic drugs.

Use caution with anticoagulants because of the risk of increased bleeding.

Monitor patients on antidiabetic drugs.

Monitor patients on antidiabetic drugs.

Don't use with alprazolam; may cause coma. Don't combine with St. John's wort, alcohol, or antidepressants; serious adverse effects can occur.

Don't combine with thyroid drugs, antihypertensives, or oral contraceptives. Will block spironolactone effects; may lead to digoxin toxicity with potassium-lowering effects.

(continued)

Precautions for herbal therapy *(continued)*

HERBAL SUBSTANCE	REPORTED USES
ma huang	*Oral:* treating colds, nasal congestion, asthma
mandrake root	*Oral:* treating fertility problems
marigold leaves or flowers	*Oral:* relieving muscle tension, increasing wound healing
melatonin	*Oral:* relieving jet lag, treating insomnia
milk thistle	*Oral:* treating hepatitis, cirrhosis, fatty liver
milk vetch	*Oral:* improving resistance to disease, adjunct therapy in chemotherapy and radiation therapy
mistletoe leaves	*Oral:* losing weight, reducing signs and symptoms of diabetes
momordica charantia	*Oral:* blocking intestinal absorption of glucose, losing weight
nettle	*Topical:* stimulating hair growth, treating bleeding *Oral:* treating rheumatism, antispasmodic, expectorant, allergic rhinitis Don't use in pregnant or breast-feeding women.
nightshade leaves or roots	*Oral:* stimulating circulatory system, treating eye disorders
octacosanol	*Oral:* treating parkinsonism, enhancing athletic performance Don't use in pregnant or breast-feeding women.
parsley seeds or leaves	*Oral:* treating jaundice, asthma, menstrual difficulties, conjunctivitis

REPORTED INTERACTIONS

Don't use with antihypertensive drugs, antidiabetic drugs, MAO inhibitors, digoxin; serious adverse effects may occur.

Monitor patients on antidiabetic drugs.

Monitor patients on antidiabetic drugs.

(continued)

Precautions for herbal therapy *(continued)*

HERBAL SUBSTANCE	REPORTED USES
passionflower vine	*Oral:* sedative/hypnotic
peppermint leaves	*Oral:* treating nervousness, insomnia, dizziness, cramps, coughs *Topical:* rubbed on forehead for relieving tension headaches
psyllium	*Oral:* treating constipation, lowering cholesterol levels
raspberry	*Oral:* healing minor wounds, controlling diabetes
red clover	*Oral:* relieving symptoms of menopause, PMS
rose hips	*Oral:* laxative, boosting the immune system and preventing illness
rosemary	*Topical:* relieving rheumatism, sprains, wounds, bruises, eczema *Oral:* gastric stimulation, relieving flatulence, stimulating bile release, relieving colic
rue extract	*Topical:* relieving pain associated with sprains, groin pulls, whiplash
saffron	*Oral:* treating menstrual problems, abortifacient
sage	*Oral:* lowering blood pressure, blood glucose
SAMe	*Oral:* promoting general health and sense of well-being
sarsaparilla	*Oral:* treating skin disorders, rheumatism

REPORTED INTERACTIONS

Risk of increased sedation with other central nervous system (CNS) depressants and MAO inhibitors. Don't use alcohol while on this drug.

Don't use with warfarin, digoxin, or lithium. Don't combine with laxatives. Monitor patients on cholesterol-lowering drugs.

Monitor patients on antidiabetic drugs.

Don't combine with heparin or warfarin because of the risk of increased bleeding. Don't combine with HRT or oral contraceptives because of the risk of increased estrogenic effects.

Don't combine with HRT or oral contraceptives.

Monitor patients on antidiabetic or antihypertensive drugs.

(continued)

Precautions for herbal therapy *(continued)*

HERBAL SUBSTANCE	REPORTED USES
sassafras	*Topical:* treating local pain, skin eruptions *Oral:* enhancing athletic performance, "curing" syphilis Oil has been toxic to fetus when ingested by children and adults.
saw palmetto	*Oral:* treating benign prostatic hypertrophy
schisandra	*Oral:* health tonic, protecting liver; adjunct in cancer chemotherapy and radiation therapy. Don't use in pregnant women.
spirulina	*Oral:* enhancing athletic performance, improving energy and boosting metabolism May be very toxic to children and pets.
squaw vine	*Oral:* diuretic, tonic, aid in labor and childbirth, treating menstrual problems
St. John's wort	*Oral:* treating depression, PMS; antiviral *Topical:* treating puncture wounds, insect bites
sweet violet flowers	*Oral:* treating respiratory disorders, emetic
tarragon	*Oral:* losing weight, lowering blood glucose, preventing cancer
thyme	*Topical:* liniment, treating wounds, gargle *Oral:* antidiarrheal, relieving bronchitis and laryngitis
turmeric	*Oral:* antioxidant, anti-inflammatory

REPORTED INTERACTIONS

Don't use with HRT or oral contraceptives. Don't combine with finasteride; serious adverse effects may occur.

Blocks vitamin B_{12} absorption.

Don't combine with drugs known to cause liver toxicity. Use caution with HRT and oral contraceptives.

Serious drug reactions reported with selective serotonin reuptake inhibitors (SSRIs), MAO inhibitors, kava, digoxin, oral contraceptives, theophylline, and AIDS/antiviral agents; avoid these combinations. Severe phototoxicity can occur if combined with other drugs that cause photosensitivity. Hypertensive crisis possible if combined with tyramine-containing foods.

Monitor patients on antidiabetic drugs.

Serious photosensitivity reactions may occur if combined with other drugs that cause photosensitivity. Don't combine with MAO inhibitors or SSRIs; serious adverse effects have been noted.

Don't use with anticoagulants because of the risk of increased bleeding.

(continued)

Precautions for herbal therapy (continued)

HERBAL SUBSTANCE	REPORTED USES
valerian	*Oral:* sedative/hypnotic, reducing anxiety, relaxing muscles
went rice	*Oral:* cholesterol-lowering Don't use in pregnant or breast-feeding women, in alcoholics, or in patients with known liver disease.
white willow bark	*Oral:* treating fevers
wild yam	*Oral:* enhancing athletic performance, increasing energy and sense of well-being Causes estrogenic effects.
xuan seng	*Oral:* lowering blood glucose, slowing heart rate, treating heart failure
yohimbe	*Oral:* treating erectile dysfunction

er methods. The patient, thinking that these are just "natural" products, may feel that this is a harmless additional therapy that helps his condition. In many cases, the patient doesn't report the use of herbal therapies because he doesn't think of them as drugs or as something that could be detrimental to his health or disrupt his medical regimen. The patient may feel that his health care provider may not approve of these remedies, so he doesn't mention them to avoid conflict. (See *Problems with herbal therapy,* page 90.)

REPORTED INTERACTIONS

Don't use with barbiturates, alcohol, CNS depressants, or antihistamines; serious sedation may occur. Use caution with other drugs known to cause liver toxicity.

Don't combine with other drugs known to cause liver toxicity.

Don't combine with alcohol, metrondiazole, HRT, or oral contraceptives.

Monitor patients on antidiabetic drugs.

Monitor patients on antihypertensive drugs, beta blockers, and anticholinergic drugs.

PREVENT IT

Medication error: Janet Gibbs, a 43-year-old school teacher, was feeling very sad, lethargic, and depressed. After an evaluation, her health care provider prescribed citalopram (Celexa), a selective serotonin reuptake inhibitor (SSRI) antidepressant. At her 6-week evaluation, Janet was feeling much better. She reported that she was able to get up each morning and go to work. She said she felt confident again and no longer described herself as depressed. Two weeks later, Janet called her health care provider with complaints of sweating, flushed skin, headache, palpitations, and nausea. She was seen that day for evaluation. While talking with the

Problems with herbal therapy

The public now has many natural substances available for self-treating many complaints. These substances, the use of which is derived from folklore and medical traditions of various cultures, commonly have identified ingredients with known therapeutic activities. Some of these substances have unknown mechanisms of action, but over the years have been reliably used to relieve specific symptoms. Some may contain unknown ingredients, which may one day prove useful in modern pharmacology.

Because herbal products aren't subject to the long evaluation process that's required for traditional drugs, the actual effects of many of these products may not be known. Available scientific information may be based on a very limited number of cases.

Another problem that may arise with the use of herbal products is the lack of quality control over many products. It has been found that the actual active component in these products may vary among batches and manufacturers. A patient may switch brands and experience different effects. Studies have shown that because many of these products are ground roots, leaves, or flowers, the potency varies depending on the time of year, the plant's water supply, the fertilizer used, and the harvesting process. The patient needs advice on what active ingredients to look for, what other ingredients to be aware of, and how to gauge the recommended dose of these products.

The real danger is that some herbal substances can compromise conventional medical treatment or even cause life-threatening effects. As the use of these products increases, the incidence of reported adverse effects and drug interactions is also increasing.

If a patient reports using an herbal substance, check the reported uses for an indication of potential interactions with prescription drugs. For example, if a patient reports using false unicorn root to ease menopause symptoms, know that this product may dramatically alter the expected effect of hormone replacement therapy or estrogen receptor modulators.

nurse, she mentioned how frustrated she was with the depression. She had been feeling so much better that she was becoming active, beginning an exercise program, and starting a healthy lifestyle campaign. When asked about the healthy lifestyle campaign, Janet reported that she had begun taking St. John's wort — a product she had seen advertised on television that was supposed to alleviate depression "naturally." She thought she might be able to stop taking drugs if she could alleviate her depression in another way. Reviewing St. John's wort, the nurse discovered that it shouldn't be taken with SSRIs because of the risk of severe reactions. Janet was asked to stop the St. John's wort and monitor her reaction.

Prevention: *Janet Gibbs was in a situation familiar to many consumers who want to turn to natural treatments to control their problems. These products, however, act as drugs in the body. When a patient is prescribed a drug (such as warfarin, SSRIs, diabetic drugs, anticoagulants, oral contraceptives, or antiviral drugs) that has documented interactions with herbal therapies, she should receive written information about the need to report the use of herbal products and the potential for interactions with these products. The information needs to be shared in a nonjudgmental manner and should become a routine part of patient-teaching programs. Janet could have prevented her reaction if she had known that she should avoid St. John's wort.*

Although patients commonly feel that herbal products are "natural" and therefore benign, research on some herbal products has turned up decided problems with their use. The problems are inherent in the herbs and don't stem from concomitant use with conventional drugs or OTC products.

PREVENT IT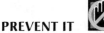

Medication error: *George Davis arrived at the clinic with complaints of fatigue, easy bruising, swelling in his legs, and indigestion. He had no known medical problems, and a complete physical examination revealed a low-grade fever, blood* *pressure of 150/92 mm Hg, a pulse rate of 88, a respiratory rate of 24, an enlarged liver, and slightly yellow sclera. Blood tests revealed elevated levels of hepatic enzyme. Mr. Davis denied alcohol or drug use and stated that he didn't take medications. While talking with the nurse about other medications, his wife mentioned that he had been drinking comfrey tea because of a chronic upset stomach. He didn't want to use OTC drugs and had read that comfrey was soothing for upset stomachs. As his workup for liver dysfunction continued, the nurse researched comfrey. She discovered that this product was associated with liver damage, bladder tumors, various cancers, and veno-occlusive disease. It was decided to pursue the comfrey as the main factor in his liver problems.*

__Prevention:__ The FDA has sent a warning letter to producers of herbal products that contain comfrey stating that it has been determined that comfrey isn't safe if ingested and should be removed from the market. Comfrey, which contains pyrolizidine alkaloids, has been associated with liver damage and other serious adverse effects. Although there are no scientific data on its effectiveness, it's reportedly used to treat various internal ailments, from ulcers to liver and gallbladder disease. Comfrey is commonly prepared as a tea to soothe upset stomachs. The herb is commercially available as common comfrey, prickly comfrey, and Russian comfrey. Producers and distributors of products containing comfrey have been advised to recall the products or face direct enforcement action.

Patients known to use herbal remedies and alternative therapies should be alerted to the potential dangers associated with this herbal product. Mr. Davis thought he was taking the sensible and "natural" approach to treating his chronically upset stomach. He delayed seeking medical attention and may well have caused liver damage by using this herbal remedy. Education is the best prevention for this type of problem. The alert nurse asked the right questions and discovered the source of the problem.

With the growing use of herbal remedies and alternative therapies, concern continues to build about the lack of regulation and standardization in this industry. These products are considered to be dietary supplements and aren't subject to intense scrutiny. Consequently, the amount of herb may vary from product to product, and the product may contain questionable additives.

PREVENT IT

Medication error: Janice Howell's diabetes has been well regulated with metformin/glyburide (Glucovance), diet, and exercise. She has discussed her desire to use herbal products with her health care provider and has been using ginseng to improve her memory and sense of well-being. Her medical regimen was established while she was using ginseng, and she was asked to notify her health care provider if anything changed in her use pattern for ginseng or if she added other herbal therapies. Over the past 2 weeks, she has been experiencing dizziness accompanied by sweating, heart palpitations, and feelings of anxiety. Her home blood glucose checks have been lower than her normal. She came in for evaluation, and her diet, exercise, and drug regimen was reviewed. Nothing seemed to have changed with her drug, diet, and exercise regimen, and she had no sign of infection or other problems. Discussing her program, Janice remembered that she had started using a new, less-expensive brand of ginseng. She said that the package stated that it contained the same active ingredient and recommended the same dose. Because ginseng is known to cause hypoglycemia when combined with diabetic agents, the thinking was that the new brand of ginseng actually contained more ginseng per dose than the old brand, leading to the patient's hypoglycemic episodes.

Prevention: Ginseng is a popular product containing the active ingredients ginsenosides and eleuthreosides. It's used to *improve cognitive function, stamina and healing, and well-being; it's also used as an aphrodisiac. The American Journal of Clinical Nutrition reported a random assay of 25 commercial ginseng products. Although the 25 products reviewed were all found to have accurate labels, a significant variability in the amount of active product was noted. There was a 15-fold concentration variation in the actual ginsenoside content and a 43-fold variation in the actual eleuthoroside concentration. Of the 11 products that listed the content of active ingredients on their labels, six were found to have less ginseng than the label stated and five were found to have more than the label stated. This random study points out the problems that can be encountered with the herbal or "natural" therapies being widely advertised and used. After researching this, it was discovered that there can be quite a variation in actual ingredients with these products.*

Patients need to be warned about the lack of regulation and standardization in the industry, variations in product quality, and the potential for adverse effects when using these products. Also, patients who are comfortable with using one product need to be aware of the problems that could occur if they switch to a different brand of the same product. If their medical regimen is balanced around the use of a particular herbal remedy, switching brands can imbalance the effects of the medical regimen.

Routine medications

When taking a drug history, always ask the patient about the use of other medications. Although most patients immediately report other prescription drugs, they may forget to mention those that they take routinely.

Medications taken every day may be involved in drug-drug interactions and may cause potentially harmful reactions. When asking the patient about the use of OTC medications or herbal therapies, it's a good idea to also inquire about other drugs that he takes routinely. The patient is typically surprised to suddenly remember he also takes these medications. In a facility, health care providers have control over the medications being given each day and know about these types of drugs. During the admission drug history, it's very important to ask about these daily drugs so that possible drug-drug interactions can be avoided and the patient can continue on these daily therapies, if appropriate. When a patient is seen in the outpatient setting, always ask at each visit about other medications he's taking every day.

PREVENT IT

Medication error: *Gina Carl, age 44, was admitted to the emergency department (ED) with a painful and swollen foot that turned out to be a case of acute gout. Serum urate levels were elevated, and the attending physician ordered colchicine 0.6 mg P.O. followed by 0.6 mg/hour for the episode. The patient was also given a prescription for allopurinol (Zyloprim) 100 mg P.O. twice daily to avert future gout attacks. When the admitting nurse asked the patient about other medications she took, Gina stated that she took ibuprofen 600 mg for pain. When the attack had resolved and the patient was leaving, she asked the nurse if allopurinol could cause diarrhea. Gina then explained her 25-year history of Crohn's disease and reported that she takes mercaptopurine (Purinethol) 50 mg every morning with several vitamins and minerals. She didn't think to report this, stating that she didn't regard these as medications — it was just what she did every morning. In researching the drug, the nurse discovered that when allopurinol is taken concurrently with mercaptopurine, increases in mercaptopurine levels can occur, leading to serious toxic effects. The nurse also discovered that mercaptopurine can precipitate gout attacks because it can cause hyperurice-*

mia. The patient's daily drug could have contributed to her acute gout attack. If the prescribed drug had been taken with mercaptopurine, the patient could have become seriously ill.

Prevention: *The alert nurse was able to avert a potentially serious problem when the routine drug was discovered. The physician was notified, and the dosage of the mercaptopurine was decreased to 12.5 mg/day. The patient was asked to return for follow-up later in the week.*

The patient taking routine drugs — such as this one taking mercaptopurine for 25 years or a patient taking oral contraceptives or hormone replacement therapy for life — commonly forgets to mention these drugs when asked. If a patient takes a drug with a small margin of safety or one that's known to interact with many other drugs, it might be advisable to suggest that he carry or wear medical identification. Ask the patient to make a list of his medications and carry it with him for use by emergency medical personnel. When taking a drug history, always ask specifically if the patient is taking medications every day, and even list a few examples — birth control pills and thyroid or asthma medications.

Lay persons aren't the only patients who forget to mention drugs that are taken routinely. Fellow health care professionals may make this mistake, too. Always ask the patient about his use of daily medications, even if the patient happens to be a colleague.

PREVENT IT

Medication error: *Nancy Murphy, 26, is a nurse who's studying full time to become a nurse practitioner. She moved to a northeastern city to attend graduate school and, a few weeks later, developed a sinus infection. Nancy went to the University Health Service and was prescribed tetracycline.*

She was reassured that sinusitis was common in that area at that time of year, and that the 5-day antibiotic course should treat the infection. She denied having allergies or taking medications. Twelve weeks later, she returned complaining of nausea, anorexia, fluid retention, and rather uncomfortable constipation. On examination, it was discovered that Nancy was about 12 weeks' pregnant. She didn't believe the diagnosis because she was very careful about taking her birth control pills. In reviewing her chart, it was determined that Nancy probably became pregnant during the time she was taking tetracycline. The Health Service staff told Nancy that they were surprised that as a nurse she didn't know that tetracycline may affect birth control pills and that a barrier form of contraception should be used while taking that drug. Nancy then realized that, as a critical care unit nurse, she had little interaction with people using birth control pills. Her main concern now was what effect her continued use of birth control pills for the last 12 weeks had had on her baby.

Prevention: *When patients are also health care workers, it's sometimes assumed that they know what to ask and how to respond. Nancy's problem might have been prevented if she had been asked specific questions about the use of other drugs — OTC, herbal, daily, or prescribed. Nancy stated that she felt so awful when she was first seen that she just wasn't thinking clearly. She desperately wanted something to treat the sinus pain, which was the predominant thought on her mind. She had been using birth control pills for many years and it just didn't occur to her to mention these when asked about the use of other drugs. Nancy underwent several prenatal tests and, luckily, her baby was born without the possible defects that have been associated with the use of birth control pills or antibiotics during pregnancy. It's important to remember that no matter who your patient is — even a nurse or physician — you should ask specific questions about the use of other drugs.*

In today's mobile society, it's also important to ask about the use of other daily drugs even if you think you know all about a patient's medical regimen. Many patients see more than one health care provider for various reasons — a primary care provider, an allergist, a gynecologist — and these providers don't always communicate effectively with each other. Patients may assume that all of their care and information is coordinated in a central place, but that isn't always true. Asking a few questions can prevent a serious problem from occurring.

PREVENT IT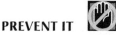

Medication error: *Pat Cameron, age 76, has chronic heart failure related to rheumatic heart disease that she had when she was a child. Her medications include digoxin (Lanoxin), furosemide (Lasix), and a potassium supplement. She's a cheerful and pleasant woman and has been coming to the clinic two times a month for the past 2 years for monitoring. After she failed to appear for a routine visit, the concerned staff discovered that she had been hospitalized with cardiac arrhythmias and hypokalemia. A staff member visited her in the hospital and talked with her about her medical care in an attempt to discover what went wrong after 2 years of successful treatment. The discussion revealed that Ms. Cameron went to several clinics each month, at least once or twice per week. All the providers at these various clinics were treating her heart failure with essentially the same therapy. Ms. Cameron had never mentioned the other clinics or prescriptions to her providers. Because she had her prescriptions filled at the pharmacies at each clinic, the duplication wasn't noted. Visiting the clinics was an important part of her socialization — she got out of the office, she knew so many nice people, and she felt that each one was doing a great job taking care of her. She took the digoxin prescribed by the clinics on the days that* *she would have gone to each clinic—blue bottle digoxin on Monday, yellow bottle digoxin on Tuesday, and so forth. When her furosemide spilled, she had put it all in one big bottle; she usually took two or three pills, depending on what she could remember about the pills on a given day. She said she didn't like her "shaking" medication—which turned out to be the potassium supplement that she took only when she felt shaky, sometimes three or four pills if she was really shaky. The shaking must have been related to hypokalemia, and she was able to stay on top of that problem with the potassium supplements. With this faulty administration method, it was amazing that toxic drug effects hadn't shown up long before 2 years.*

Prevention: Pat Cameron recovered, and her various clinics shared their records to avoid duplicating prescriptions and possible problems that could occur with taking too many of these drugs. Although she still visited her clinics, one provider now managed her drug regimen. She stated that no one ever asked her if she was seeing another physician or had other prescriptions. Everyone assumed that they knew the patient; each group had the medical record and could refer to it as needed. Thus, when taking a drug history, always ask a patient if he's taking other drugs—prescription, OTC, herbal remedies, or daily medications that were prescribed elsewhere.

Drugs and pregnancy

Because of the potential for adverse effects on the fetus associated with many drugs, it's important to know if a woman of childbearing years is pregnant or planning on becoming pregnant when drug therapy is started. (See *Drugs, pregnancy, and contraception,* page 100.)

Drugs, pregnancy, and contraception

A drug may be contraindicated during pregnancy because of its reported adverse effects on the fetus. Certain drugs should be used during pregnancy only when the benefit to the mother clearly outweighs the potential risk to the fetus. However, prescribers should first investigate other drugs for a possible replacement.

If the patient is *not* pregnant and *is* using oral contraceptives, however, it's important for them to know that some drugs interact with oral contraceptives and that pregnancy may result. These patients need to be informed that they should use a barrier form of contraception when receiving such drug therapy.

PREVENT IT

Medication error: *Lorraine Beasley, age 49, visited her health care provider following a cholesterol check at her local grocery store. The machine at the store reported that she should see her health care provider. Lorraine stated that she was probably perimenopausal and, because her family had a history of myocardial infarction and heart disease, she wanted to make sure that her cholesterol level was being monitored. She's an active woman who works out at a health club three times a week and follows a healthy diet. Even so, her lipid levels were quite elevated and she was started on atorvastatin (Lipitor). Three weeks later, Lorraine was admitted to the ED with acute abdominal pain and vaginal bleeding. She had a miscarriage of a fetus that was approximately 12 weeks' gestation. Although the exact cause of the miscarriage was unknown, questions were raised about the use of ator-*

vastatin, a drug in the pregnancy category X because of its known adverse effects on a fetus. Lorraine had had no idea that she was pregnant when she visited her health care provider; she thought that she was irregular because she was beginning menopause. The health care provider, when told that Lorraine thought she was perimenopausal, didn't question her further about the possibility of pregnancy.

__Prevention:__ This situation might have been avoided if Lorraine's health care provider had asked her specifically about the possibility of pregnancy. If she had said she didn't think so, she could have had a pregnancy test quickly performed in the office. Although the drug may not have caused the miscarriage, Lorraine will always wonder. Although there aren't many drugs that are in pregnancy category X, if you work in an area that uses any of these drugs, it's important to keep that in mind when taking a patient's history. Most drugs come with cautions about use during pregnancy. It's good practice to ask a woman of childbearing age if she is, could be, or is planning to become pregnant. This information will prompt the health care provider to check on a drug's pregnancy category and select another drug if that's appropriate or to include important information about contraception that might be needed with certain drugs. This was a situation in which the rule "When in doubt, check it out" could have prevented this situation.

✦ Replay: The first right

The first right in the common-sense approach to preventing medication errors is to make sure that you're treating the right patient. (See *Checklist for the right patient,* page 102.) This involves always checking the identification of the patient. Don't rely on room numbers, bed numbers, diagnoses, or your own memory. Always check a patient's ID before giving a drug.

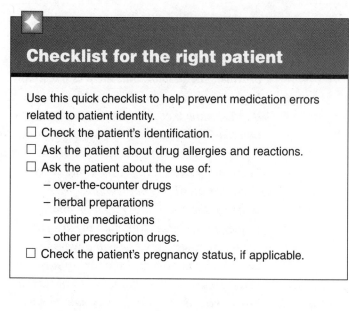

Checklist for the right patient

Use this quick checklist to help prevent medication errors related to patient identity.
☐ Check the patient's identification.
☐ Ask the patient about drug allergies and reactions.
☐ Ask the patient about the use of:
  – over-the-counter drugs
  – herbal preparations
  – routine medications
  – other prescription drugs.
☐ Check the patient's pregnancy status, if applicable.

Further, always check to make sure that the patient isn't allergic to the drug to be administered. Double-check that the patient isn't taking other prescription or OTC drugs, herbal therapies, or routine medications that could cause problems with this drug. Assure yourself about the patient's pregnancy status if she's a woman of childbearing age. Although this may sound complicated, running through a quick mental checklist before giving a drug can prevent a medication error.

Chapter

The right drug

The second "right" to consider before administering a drug is whether it's the "right drug." This means that you must ensure that the drug you're going to give is the drug that was ordered for the patient and that it was stored and prepared correctly. It also means that you must verify that the drug prescribed makes sense for that patient — is it appropriate for the condition that's being treated?

✦ The name game

Making sure that the drug you're going to give is the drug intended for the patient may be complicated by several communication challenges. "When in doubt, check it out" can be extremely important if you have difficulty understanding what was written, said, or intended. Reported problems include similar drug names, illegible handwriting, poor verbal skills, and confusing or even bogus telephone orders.

Drug names that look and sound alike

The Food and Drug Administration (FDA) has become increasingly aware of the problems that can occur with look-alike and sound-alike drug names.

IT'S A FACT

*After many errors occurred involving confusion between am-
rinone (a cardiotonic drug used to treat heart failure) and
amiodarone (an antiarrhythmic drug), the FDA requested
that the first drug's name be changed. In 2000, amrinone
was officially changed to inamrinone.*

The list of confusing drug names is long. If you work
in an area where these frequently confused drugs are
used, it's a good idea to post an alert in the medication
room, the nurses' station, or even in the break room.
Awareness of a potential problem can help to prevent
an error. (See *Commonly confused drug names.*)

IT'S A FACT

*The FDA has received 22 reports of confusion between Lamic-
tal (lamotrigine), an anticonvulsant, and Lamisil (terbinafine), and antifungal agent. As a result, patients have suffered
adverse effects, including potentially life-threatening seizures.
Recently, GlaxoSmithKline informed physicians and pharmacists of the frequent dispensing errors that have occurred
when Lamictal is prescribed; the prescription drugs most commonly confused with Lamictal are Lamisil, lamivudine, Lu-
diomil, labetalol, and Lomotil.*

Pharmacies are also busy places where medication
errors can and do occur.

(Text continues on page 113.)

✦ Commonly confused drug names

DRUG NAME	COMMONLY CONFUSED WITH
acetazolamide	acetohexamide
Aciphex (rabeprazole)	Aricept (donepezil)
alprazolam	lorazepam
Altace (ramipril)	alteplase
Altace (ramipril)	Artane (trihexyphenidyl)
alteplase	Altace (ramipril)
amantadine	rimantadine
Ambien (zolpidem)	Amen (medroxyprogesterone)
Amen (medroxyprogesterone)	Ambien (zolpidem)
amiodarone	inamrinone
Apresoline (hydralazine)	Priscoline (tolazoline)
Aricept (donepezil)	Aciphex (rabeprazole)
Artane (trihexyphenidyl)	Altace (ramipril)
bepridil	Prepidil (dinoprostone)
Brethine (terbutaline)	Brevital (methohexital)
Brevital (methohexital)	Brethine (terbutaline)
Cardene (nicardipine)	codeine
Cardura (doxazosin)	Ridaura (auranofin)
Celebrex (celecoxib)	Celexa (citalopram)

(continued)

Commonly confused drug names (continued)

DRUG NAME	COMMONLY CONFUSED WITH
Celebrex (celecoxib)	Cerebyx (fosphenytoin)
Celebrex (celecoxib)	Xanax (alprazolam)
Celexa (citalopram)	Celebrex (celecoxib)
Celexa (citalopram)	Cerebyx (fosphenytoin)
Celexa (citalopram)	Xanax (alprazolam)
Cerebyx (fosphenytoin)	Celebrex (celecoxib)
Cerebyx (fosphenytoin)	Celexa (citalopram)
Cerebyx (fosphenytoin)	Xanax (alprazolam)
chlorpromazine	chlorpropamide
chlorpropamide	chlorpromazine
clonidine	Klonopin (clonazepam)
Clozaril (clozapine)	Colazal (balsalazide)
codeine	Cardene (nicardipine)
codeine	Lodine (etodolac)
Colazal (balsalazide)	Clozaril (clozapine)
Cytosar (cytarabine)	Cytoxan (cyclophosphamide)
Cytotec (misoprostol)	Cytoxan (cyclophosphamide)
Cytoxan (cyclophosphamide)	Cytosar (cytarabine)
Cytoxan (cyclophosphamide)	Cytotec (misoprostol)

Commonly confused drug names *(continued)*

DRUG NAME	COMMONLY CONFUSED WITH
Depakote (valproic acid)	Depakote ER (valproic acid)
Depakote ER (valproic acid)	Depakote (valproic acid)
DiaBeta (glyburide)	Zebeta (bisoprolol)
Diamox (acetazolamide)	Dymelor (acetohexamide)
Diamox (acetazolamide)	Trimox (amoxicillin)
Digibind (digoxin immune fab)	DigiFab (digoxin immune fab)
DigiFab (digoxin immune fab)	Digibind (digoxin immune fab)
Edecrin (ethacrynic acid)	Eulexin (flutamide)
esomeprazole	omeprazole
Eulexin (flutamide)	Edecrin (ethacrynic acid)
fentanyl	sufentanil
folic acid	folinic acid
folinic acid	folic acid
Fosamax (alendronate)	Flomax (tamsulosin)
furosemide	torsemide
Hycodan (hydrocodone)	Vicodin (hydrocodone/acetaminophen)
hydralazine	hydroxyzine
hydroxyzine	hydralazine

(continued)

Commonly confused drug names *(continued)*

DRUG NAME	COMMONLY CONFUSED WITH
inamrinone	amiodarone
Inderal (propranolol)	Toradol (ketorolac)
Inversine (mecamylamine)	Invirase (saquinavir)
Invirase (saquinavir)	Inversine (mecamylamine)
iodine	Lodine (etodolac)
Isordil (isosorbide)	Plendil (felodipine)
Klonopin (clonazepam)	clonidine
Lamictal (lamotrigine)	Lamisil (terbinafine)
Lamictal (lamotrigine)	Lomotil (diphenoxylate/atropine)
Lamisil (terbinafine)	Lamictal (lamotrigine)
Lantus (insulin glargine)	Lente (insulin)
Lente (insulin)	Lantus (insulin glargine)
leucovorin	Leukeran (chlorambucil)
Leukeran (chlorambucil)	leucovorin
Libritabs (chlordiazepoxide)	Librium (chlordiazepoxide)
Librium (chlordiazepoxide)	Libritabs (chlordiazepoxide)
Lodine (etodolac)	codeine
Lodine (etodolac)	iodine
Lomotil (diphenoxylate/atropine)	Lamictal (lamotrigine)

Commonly confused drug names (continued)

DRUG NAME	COMMONLY CONFUSED WITH
Loniten (minoxidil)	Lotensin (benazepril)
Lopurin (allopurinol)	Lupron (leuprolide)
lorazepam	alprazolam
Lotensin (benazepril)	Loniten (minoxidil)
Lupron (leuprolide)	Lopurin (allopurinol)
Lupron (leuprolide)	Nuprin (ibuprofen)
Nuprin (ibuprofen)	Lupron (leuprolide)
Occlusal-HP (salicyclic acid)	Ocuflox (oxafloxacin)
Ocufen (flurbiprofen)	Ocuflox (oxafloxacin)
Ocuflox (oxafloxacin)	Ocufen (flurbiprofen)
Ocuflox (oxafloxacin)	Occlusal-HP (salicyclic acid)
omeprazole	esomeprazole
Parlodel (bromocriptine)	pindolol
Paxil (paroxetine)	Taxol (paclitaxel)
pindolol	Parlodel (bromocriptine)
pindolol	Plendil (felodipine)
Plendil (felodipine)	Isordil (isosorbide)
Plendil (felodipine)	pindolol
Plendil (felodipine)	Prinivil (lisinopril)

(continued)

Commonly confused drug names *(continued)*

DRUG NAME	COMMONLY CONFUSED WITH
Prepidil (dinoprostone)	bepridil
Prilosec (omeprazole)	Prozac (fluoxetine)
Prinivil (lisinopril)	Plendil (felodipine)
Prinivil (lisinopril)	Proventil (albuterol)
Priscoline (tolazoline)	Apresoline (hydralazine)
probenecid	Procanbid (procainamide)
Procan SR (procainamide)	Procanbid (procanamide)
Procanbid (procainamide)	probenecid
Procanbid (procainamide)	Procan SR (procainamide)
Proscar (finasteride)	Prozac (fluoxetine)
Prostin 15 (carboprost; Europe)	Prostin E_2 (dinoprostone)
Prostin 15 (carboprost; Europe)	Prostin F (dinoprost; non-USA)
Prostin 15 (carboprost; Europe)	Prostin VR Pediatric (alprostadil)
Prostin E_2 (dinoprostone)	Prostin 15 (carboprost; Europe)
Prostin E_2 (dinoprostone)	Prostin F (dinoprost; non-USA)
Prostin E_2 (dinoprostone)	Prostin VR Pediatric (alprostadil)
Prostin F (dinoprost; non-USA)	Prostin 15 (carboprost; Europe)
Prostin F (dinoprost; non-USA)	Prostin E_2 (dinoprostone)
Prostin F (dinoprost; non-USA)	Prostin VR Pediatric (alprostadil)

Commonly confused drug names *(continued)*

DRUG NAME	COMMONLY CONFUSED WITH
Prostin VR Pediatric (alprostadil)	Prostin 15 (carboprost; Europe)
Prostin VR Pediatric (alprostadil)	Prostin E$_2$ (dinoprostone)
Prostin VR Pediatric (alprostadil)	Prostin F (dinoprost; non-USA)
Proventil (albuterol)	Prinivil (lisinopril)
Prozac (fluoxetine)	Proscar (finasteride)
Retrovir (zidovudine)	ritonavir
Ridaura (auranofin)	Cardura (doxazosin)
rifabutin	rifampin
rifampin	rifabutin
rimantadine	amantadine
ritonavir	Retrovir (zidovudine)
saquinavir	Sinequan (doxepin)
Sarafem (fluoxetine)	Serophene (clomiphene)
Serophene (clomiphene)	Sarafem (fluoxetine)
Sinequan (doxepin)	saquinavir
sufentanil	fentanyl
tacrine	Tequin (gatifloxacin)
Taxol (paclitaxel)	Taxotere (docetaxel)
Taxol (paclitaxel)	Paxil (paroxetine)

(continued)

Commonly confused drug names *(continued)*

DRUG NAME	COMMONLY CONFUSED WITH
Taxotere (docetaxel)	Taxol (paclitaxel)
Tequin (gatifloxacin)	tacrine
Toradol (ketorolac)	tramadol
Toradol (ketorolac)	Inderal (propranolol)
torsemide	furosemide
tramadol	Toradol (ketorolac)
Trimox (amoxicillin)	Diamox (acetazolamide)
Tylox (oxycodone/acetaminophen)	Xanax (alprazolam)
VePesid (etoposide)	Versed (midazolam)
Versed (midazolam)	VePesid (etoposide)
Vicodin (hydrocodone/acetaminophen)	Hycodan (hydrocodone)
Vioxx (rofecoxib)	Zyvox (linezolid)
Viracept (nelfinavir)	Viramune (nevirapine)
Viramune (nevirapine)	Viracept (nelfinavir)
Xanax (alprazolam)	Zantac (ranitidine)
Xanax (alprazolam)	Celebrex (celecoxib)
Xanax (alprazolam)	Celexa (citalopram)
Xanax (alprazolam)	Cerebyx (fosphenytoin)

Commonly confused drug names *(continued)*

DRUG NAME	COMMONLY CONFUSED WITH
Xanax (alprazolam)	Tylox (oxycodone/acetaminophen)
Zantac (ranitidine)	Xanax (alprazolam)
Zantac (ranitidine)	Zyrtec (cetirizine)
Zebeta (bisoprolol)	DiaBeta (glyburide)
Zyprexa (olanzapine)	Zyrtec (cetirizine)
Zyrtec (cetirizine)	Zantac (ranitidine)
Zyrtec (cetirizine)	Zyprexa (olanzapine)
Zyvox (linezolid)	Vioxx (rofecoxib)

PREVENT IT

Medication error: A patient taking cetirizine (Zyrtec), an antihistamine, picked up a refill prescription at his local pharmacy. This pharmacy had been affected by the shortage of pharmacists in the area, and the staff was pressured with work. At home, the patient started taking pills from the new bottle. Within a short period, he felt dizzy, light-headed, and nauseated and went to bed. His wife became concerned when he slept for almost 18 hours, and the next day she called his health care provider. Because the patient had a long history of heart failure and other coronary problems, the health care provider was concerned and asked him to come in immediately. The patient was in the habit of bringing all of his medications every time he saw the health care provider, and the nurse practitioner always reviewed them with him. Because he hadn't taken any of his pills that day, the nurse used the opportunity to evaluate his knowledge of his medications while he took his drugs. The patient noticed that the pills in his Zyrtec bottle looked very different from the patient's usual pills, something he hadn't realized the day before. They checked the code number on one pill and discovered that the bottle was full of olanzapine (Zyprexa) tablets. This antipsychotic drug is associated with central nervous system (CNS) effects, including dizziness and nervousness, and cardiovascular effects, such as hypotension and tachycardia. Upon investigation, the pharmacy discovered that a drug name error (Zyrtec/Zyprexa) had occurred while the overworked pharmacist was filling the prescription. Both drugs are available in 5- and 10-mg forms and were stocked alphabetically in the pharmacy.

Prevention: *The Institute for Safe Medication Practices (ISMP) indicates that this mix-up has been reported several times in the past. Because this name confusion is known, it's important that all health care providers who prescribe, dispense, or administer these drugs remain on alert to the potential for errors. Luckily, this patient only took one does of Zyprexa and was at home when the adverse effects occurred. Although he wasn't harmed, the situation could have been different if he had been driving his car or in a vulnerable position when the dizziness and light-headedness occurred. Pharmacies have been urged to post the names of look-alike drugs with error potential on their computers and in their stock rooms. They're also advised not to store these drugs near each other.*

To help prevent errors, prescribers are urged to include generic and brand names on prescriptions as well as the indications for the drugs. Patients should be taught to look carefully at and verify the identity of the drugs they're given and to understand why these drugs have been prescribed.

Nurses, who are often the last check in the system, should ask specifically for the generic and brand names when receiving an order and should check the indications for the drug. They also should ask patients the names of the drugs and indications when administering the drugs, and use the opportunity to teach patients about their drug regimens. If patients question a particular drug, the nurse should use the opportunity to verify the drug and the order. Patients who've been using a particular drug may be much more familiar with its appearance and use than a busy nurse giving out medications. When in doubt, check it out.

Label errors

Check that label! Some labels, like some drug names, are very similar. When reading a label, first check the generic name, which is a simplified form of the drug's chemical name. Then note the trade (brand) name. Then compare both to the order that was given and make sure that they match before giving the drug. (See *Avoiding label confusion,* page 116.)

IT'S A FACT

In February 2002, a 51-year-old Connecticut woman died because her prescription for "camphorated tincture of opium" (paregoric) was filled with "opium tincture" (morphine). She was being treated for chronic diarrhea. The dose she took contained approximately 50 mg of morphine, a toxic dose approximately 10 to 20 times the usual does for pain relief.

Poor handwriting

Physicians traditionally have been considered to have illegible handwriting. Nurses, secretaries, and pharmacists who have worked with prescriptions and orders

✦ Avoiding label confusion

Don't be fooled by look-alike labels. The following labels are examples of look-alike and sound-alike names that you must read carefully to avoid medication errors.

NORPRAMIN AND NORPACE

At first glance, these medication names may easily be confused. Inadvertent substitution of the tricyclic antidepressant Norpramin for the antiarrhythmic Norpace would prevent the patient's arrhythmia from being controlled, and this could lead to serious complications.

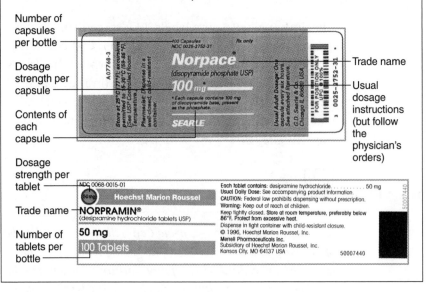

Number of capsules per bottle

Dosage strength per capsule

Contents of each capsule

Dosage strength per tablet

Trade name

Number of tablets per bottle

Trade name

Usual dosage instructions (but follow the physician's orders)

develop an amazing ability to decipher what appear, to the casual observer, to be scribbles. However, errors resulting from illegible handwriting still occur. There are three people whose handwriting may contribute to errors during the writing, transcribing, and filling of a medication order — the prescriber who writes the original prescription, the secretary or nurse who transcribes it to an order sheet, and the pharmacist who further transcribes and fills the order. All provide ample opportunity for an error to occur.

PREVENT IT

Medication error: *When the evening secretary for the medical unit called out sick, the secretary from a psychiatric unit was assigned to work in her place. Mr. Fines, age 68, was newly admitted with pneumonia, and the attending physician prescribed the antibiotic tetracycline (Sumycin) 250 mg every 6 hours. The secretary interpreted the physician's writing to be an order for the antidepressant doxepin (Sinequan). The secretary was familiar with Sinequan because it was used frequently on the psychiatric unit where she worked. Never having heard of Sumycin, she found it easy to interpret the handwriting to be something familiar: Sinequan. The nurse who checked the order didn't notice the error; in fact, when it was discovered, she pointed out how easy it was to read the order as Sinequan. The patient only received one dose of the medication before another nurse, who was familiar with both drugs, noticed that the dose ordered for Sinequan was much higher than normal. Checking through the medical record and physician orders, she discovered the error.*

Prevention: *Never assume that you can interpret another person's handwriting. When in doubt, check it out. If the secretary had contacted the attending physician or asked the nurse about the drug ordered, this error could have been prevented. It isn't uncommon for people to assume they know what something is supposed to be based on their own experience. In some facilities, prescribers are asked to write and print drug orders. This practice still doesn't guarantee that orders will be legible. Other facilities require that prescribers who are ordering a brand name drug to also include the generic name. The chances of the generic and brand names looking alike are far less likely.*

As still another check against errors, some facilities send a carbon copy to the pharmacy filling the order. This sometimes brings an error to light because the drug filled is different from the one that the nurse has in her medication Kardex.

Sometimes the prescriber has such illegible handwriting that the drugs being ordered may not seem to be even remotely related to what was actually intended. In such cases, it's always important to check with the prescriber. If you notice that the handwriting is difficult to interpret, asking for the generic and brand names is a good way to help prevent medication errors. When it comes to avoiding medication errors, never assume.

PREVENT IT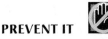

Medication error: The ISMP has reported some amazing misinterpretations of handwritten orders. Look at the order below. Decide how you would transcribe, fill, or administer the drug ordered.

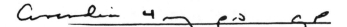

The order is for the antidiabetic agent rosiglitazone (Avandia), 4 mg orally. Most health care professionals who have looked at this order have misinterpreted it as warfarin (Coumadin), 4 mg, an anticoagulant. The order was transcribed as Coumadin, a drug familiar to many people. That familiarity commonly tricks the eye into seeing what it thinks it sees. The patient received only one dose of the wrong drug before the prescriber caught the error.

Prevention: At first glance, Avandia and Coumadin don't seem to have much in common. When you look at the prescriber's handwriting, however, it's clearly possible to make this mistake. At the time this error occurred, Avandia was a new drug most likely unfamiliar to the person reading the order. Seeing that the 4-mg dose was somewhat illegible should have alerted the reader that interpretation might be difficult. The best way to prevent misinterpretation of written orders is always to check it out. When in doubt, check it out. Don't guess; don't assume.

Verbal orders

Verbal orders always have been a source of medication errors. It isn't always possible to interpret correctly what a person is saying. As in the previous examples, interpreting what you're hearing is much like interpreting what you're seeing. If you think a person should be saying one thing, you may interpret what's being said as what you think it should be, not what it is. Working with health care professionals who have different accents or who use varying pronunciations for words, especially drug names, can add to the confusion. Most facilities have strict policies about who may take or give verbal orders and a formal policy requiring the prescriber to sign the actual order as written within a given time frame, usually 24 to 48 hours.

PREVENT IT

Medication error: The attending physician making rounds on the medical unit had a very bad head cold. He was somewhat difficult to understand and in a hurry to complete his rounds and go home. He told the nurse he wanted Mr. Foley to receive 50 mg hydralazine orally twice daily for his hypertension and heart failure. Because the nurse thought that he ordered hydroxyzine, she asked the physician to repeat the order. He did so, and she still heard him say hydroxyzine. Hy-

dralazine is a vasodilator used to treat hypertension, whereas hydroxyzine is an antihistamine and an antianxiety drug.

The secretary transcribed the order that the nurse wrote, and the physician left after saying that he would sign all of his orders in the morning. The evening nurse who checked new orders thought it was odd that a very calm patient, such as Mr. Foley, would be getting such a strong antianxiety drug. Unable to reach the attending physician, she held the evening dose of the drug with a note to check with the physician about the order. The next day, the physician came to sign his notes and corrected the error.

Prevention: *The first nurse might have been able to prevent the error if she had asked the physician to spell the name of the drug or to suggest a brand name. In this situation, the physician's illness and desire to go home might have thwarted any effort by the nurse to further clarify what was being said. Remember, the patient's safety always comes first. When you can't understand what's being said because of an accent, low voice, or nasal congestion, take the extra step to try to clarify exactly what's being said. When in doubt, check it out.*

Telephone orders

Frequently, orders are needed from a prescriber who's elsewhere. Nursing homes and long-term care facilities may need to call a prescriber for an order for a patient who can't go to an office or an acute care facility, community health care providers may need to contact a prescriber from the patient's home, and hospital nurses may need to contact attending physicians during office hours, at night, or when those providers aren't at the hospital.

Since telephone orders began, the opportunity for error has been recognized. The connection may be poor and the receiver may not understand the words clearly; also, the caller may be hurried and under stress.

IT'S A FACT

A serious overdose was reported when a telephone order for alprazolam (Xanax) 0.125 mg as needed was misinterpreted as Xanax "point 1 to 5" mg as needed.

The person taking the medication order may have been distracted by something and not listening fully to the telephone conversation. Many external factors can lead to a misinterpretation of orders. Many facilities have strict policies about who can accept telephone orders and how these orders are processed. Some facilities require that two people be on the line to verify what's being said. Many facilities require that the prescriber come in and sign the orders in person within a particular time frame — for example, within 24 or 48 hours. It's important to check your facility's policy to understand what's permitted.

PREVENT IT

Medication error: *Patricia Glenn, age 52, was admitted to a rehabilitation facility 3 days after getting a knee replacement. The order sheet that came with her stated that the staff should continue all medications she took at home. The only drugs on the medication sheet were conjugated estrogens (for menopause symptoms) and amoxicillin (for a persistent skin infection).*

Shortly after she arrived, her attending physician called to say that he wanted another medication started. He was calling from his cell phone and had a strong accent. It sounded as if he ordered Celexa (citalopram), an antidepressant, 200 mg/ day. He was asked to repeat the order, and this time it sounded as if he said Cerebyx (fosphenytoin), an antiepileptic drug.

He was asked to spell the name of the drug and he simply stated Celexa, not understanding the request. The nurse taking the order knew that Celexa was an antidepressant and asked if the patient was depressed. The physician stated that maybe she was depressed as a result of immobility, and then the cell phone connection was lost. The nurse looked up both drugs and found that the dosage for Celexa and Cerebyx was 20 mg/day. She also noted that Cerebyx was an antiepileptic drug.

Knowing that the patient didn't have seizures, the nurse decided that she must have heard the dosage wrong and wrote the order for Celexa, 20 mg/day.

Two days later, the patient mentioned that she was in considerable pain and that her mouth was extremely dry. The nurse checked her medication sheet and discovered that the patient wasn't receiving anything for pain.

When contacted, the attending physician said he was surprised that the pain medication wasn't working because it had worked so well previously. Puzzled, the nurse asked specifically which medication the patient took for pain, and the physician answered Celebrex (celecoxib), a cyclooxygenase-2 nonsteroidal anti-inflammatory drug (NSAID) 200 mg/day. The physician's telephone orders for this patient had really been misunderstood. Confusion about the drug name led to confusion about the dose, and the wrong order was written.

Prevention: *This situation was a case of multiple misunderstandings. Several measures may have prevented it. (See* Preventing verbal medication errors.*)*

Bogus orders

Over the past few years, there also have been reports of imposters calling in telephone orders. With the busy pace of most health care facilities, frequent staffing shortages, and the many health care providers who can write orders, some people have managed to "play

Preventing verbal medication errors

To help prevent errors in medication orders communicated verbally, take the following precautions.

✦ Have another person listen in on the telephone call and verify what you hear.

✦ Don't write the order for the medication unless you're certain of the order; question the prescriber and confirm the order.

✦ Ask the prescriber to give you the generic and brand names of the drug. Chances are slim that generic and brand names sound alike.

✦ Ask the prescriber the indication for which the drug is intended.

✦ Repeat what you think you heard; if you're still confused, ask the prescriber to spell the name of the drug — not all prescribers can accurately spell drug names, but your question will raise awareness of a potential error in the order.

✦ Have the prescriber come in to countersign verbal telephone orders within 24 hours.

✦ As an added check, always tell the patient what drug you're going to give them and why. If it's supposed to be a routine medication and the patient doesn't know what it is, hold the drug and verify the order.

As with any situation, "when in doubt, check it out."

doctor" and actually call in prescriptions. Strict telephone order policies are the best way to prevent this type of error. Many facilities have also had to extend their policies to encompass faxed and computer-generated orders. Technological sophistication allows some people access to patient information that should be protected. The alert nurse who asks the appropriate questions can prevent these types of errors.

Relying on drug name patterns

Commonly, drugs of a similar class have "clues" in their brand names to indicate what they are. For instance, the penicillins, a large class of antibiotic drugs, usually contain the "illin" ending in the brand name — Totacillin, Wycillin — or "pen" as a suffix — Pfizerpen, Omnipen. This isn't a rule to drug naming, however, and sometimes a penicillin doesn't contain either of these clues — for example, Veetids or Trimox. The cephalosporins all begin with "cef" or "ceph," except one: loracarbef.

Busy health professionals may become comfortable with a certain way of recognizing a drug's class because of its name. This can lead to errors when a drug doesn't fit the pattern. Again, the rule of thumb should always be "when in doubt, check it out"; don't assume you know what a drug is based on its name alone.

PREVENT IT

Medication error: *Larry Priest, a 63-year-old executive on a business trip, was admitted to the emergency department (ED) with complaints of fever, chills, agitation, and lower abdominal bloating and pain. His history was insignificant except for a penicillin allergy. On admission, his vital signs were: pulse rate, 124 beats/minute; respiration rate, 28 breaths/ minute; temperature, 103° F (39.4° C); and blood pressure, 92/56 mm Hg. He was cool, clammy, and unable to void. A urine sample, obtained by catheterization, revealed 4+ white blood cells and gross bacteria. Mr. Priest was diagnosed with urosepsis.*

The ED attending physician had just returned from a week's vacation and noted that ampicillin/sulbactam (Unasyn), a new drug for urosepsis, was being written about in the medical journals, so he ordered it: Unasyn 2 g I.V. every 6 hours. The pharmacist dispensed the drug, and the nurse administered the first dose. When Mr. Priest asked about the drug, the physician responded that it was an antibiotic for urinary infections.

Three hours after receiving the drug, the patient's condition improved; his pulse and respirations were decreased and his blood pressure increased to a normal range. When the nurse changed his gown, she noticed that he appeared to have hives on his chest and back. Further assessment revealed noisy respirations and that Mr. Priest was feeling somewhat anxious. The nurse recognized these signs and symptoms as a drug reaction. Knowing that the patient was allergic to penicillin, the nurse looked up Unasyn in a new drug guide and discovered that it's a combination antibiotic containing ampicillin (a penicillin) and sulbactam. The physician was notified, and the drug was changed to ofloxacin (Floxin). The patient was given diphenhydramine (Benadryl), an antihistamine, to counteract the effects of the allergic reaction.

Prevention: *This medication error can be explained in a few ways. Perhaps the physician wasn't expecting a penicillin because penicillins aren't usually regarded as appropriate drugs for urinary tract infections; they're typically used for respiratory or skin infections. However, this combination of ampicillin and sulbactam has proven to be very effective against many bacteria. The drug name, however, didn't have the usual clues that are found with penicillin drugs—namely, "illin" and "pen" were missing from the brand name. The write-ups for Unasyn didn't focus on the drug's ingredients, only its effectiveness. The physician only remembered that it was promoted as effective against urosepsis. Unfortunately, no one took the extra step to look up the drug. Luckily for Mr. Priest, the nurse recognized the signs of an allergic reaction, discontinued the drug, and treated the reaction. This error could have been prevented if the prescriber or the nurse had investigated the drug before prescribing or administering it. It's never a good idea to assume that you can figure out what a drug is from its name. When in doubt, check it out.*

✦ I.V. and TPN solutions

Although not technically drugs, problems can occur with I.V. and total parenteral nutrition (TPN) solutions. Always check the contents of an infusion bag before you hang it. Errors have occurred when the wrong label has been put on an I.V. bag after drugs were added. Pharmacies premix TPN solutions and label the bags. All too often, it's easy to just check the patient's name and ignore the long list of contents in the solution. The mixture should be carefully checked against the orders. Errors can happen, and patients can receive nutrients or electrolytes that may cause cardiovascular or hepatic failure. Always check the label with the order; don't assume that the pharmacy is always correct.

Unit-dose systems reduce waste by allowing facilities to reuse drugs or I.V. solutions that were ordered for a patient, but weren't used because of a change in orders or a patient discharge. However, if more than one label appears on an I.V. or TPN solution, how do you know which is correct? The best response is to avoid using a solution that seems to be mislabeled or confusing. Safety should be your primary concern.

Other problems have been reported to occur when I.V. or TPN solutions are attached to the wrong I.V. lines or access ports when they're administered. Sometimes, the patient has numerous tubes and it may be easy to connect an infusion to the wrong I.V. line. Many facilities require dedicated TPN lines and labels.

PREVENT IT

Medication error: *Bill Stout, age 72, was hospitalized following a severe bout of gastroenteritis. His potassium level was low, and a secondary potassium piggyback of 20 mEq I.V.*

was ordered for him to be infused over 4 hours. The pharmacy dispensed the medication, and the nurse started the infusion. After 30 minutes, the patient became restless and had difficulty breathing. He was started on oxygen therapy. Fortunately, it was quickly discovered that the "potassium" infusion was really penicillin, to which the patient had an allergy. Although the label on the infusion bag said potassium, the bag underneath the label was imprinted with the penicillin dose. The infusion was discontinued; the patient was treated with diphenhydramine (Benadryl), an antihistamine, and suffered no ill effects.

Prevention: Mistakes happen. The pharmacist may be extremely busy or distracted when preparing medications. The simple task of placing a label on a premixed medication infusion can still go wrong. In this case, the pharmacist placed the right label (with the patient's name) on the wrong drug. This could have been fatal for the patient if it hadn't been discovered quickly. Never assume that the label on a premixed bag of medication is correct. Be sure to check not only the label that the pharmacy placed on the bag, but also check that it's on the correct bag of medication.

✦ Computer-generated orders

Using computers to manage drug orders or the prescription process doesn't guarantee that errors won't occur. The computer can only work with the information that's entered into it. If the person reading the medication order makes a mistake in deciphering the handwriting, and then enters that misinterpretation, a medication error has occurred. Always go back to the original order when trying to verify that you're going to give the right drug, even if it was computer generated.

PREVENT IT

Medication error: A physician prescribed Cardene (nicardipine), a calcium channel blocker, 30 mg orally every 8 hours to treat hypertension in a patient who also had a history of migraine headaches. The office nurse responsible for preparing the prescriptions on a computer system knew the patient also had severe migraine headaches and read the order as codeine, 30 mg orally every 8 hours.

The patient took the prescription to the local pharmacy. The pharmacist, who had only the computer-generated signed prescription, filled it as it was written. The following day, the physician was signing laboratory values that had come in and noticed the error. When he asked the nurse about the error, she stated that she knew the patient had severe migraines and believed that a pain medication seemed appropriate; she had never heard of Cardene. Even the physician had to admit that his handwriting could easily have been misread as codeine.

Prevention: This small clinic was able to work with the physician's handwriting problems by always requiring that he provide the brand and generic names for drugs and an indication on the prescription. If this system was originally in place, the nurse would have noticed that codeine wasn't an appropriate drug of choice for treating hypertension and questioned the physician before entering the order into the computer system.

✦ Electronic or printed forms

To bypass some problems associated with illegible handwriting, misunderstood words, and the possibility of errors when many people are involved in the transcription of orders, many facilities use preprinted forms

or electronic orders and charts. These aren't total safeguards for preventing medication errors. Many people
come to rely on computers and forms and aren't nearly as careful as they are when using handwritten information.

It's easy to allow things to slide or neglect to check
on drug information when it's on a computer-generated form. It's easy to assume that someone else has
checked it out. However, it's the people who use these
forms who are responsible for accurate and safe practice. A computer form is still only as good as the person who's using it.

Many computer programs use various standards
that are known to cause problems and medication errors—for example, in almost all computer formats, if
there's a dose that uses a decimal point, all doses must
have a decimal point. If 1.5 mg is used, then 2.0 mg
will be used. Small letters and blurry computer screens
can lead to a misinterpretation of 2.0 as 20. This could
cause an error of 10-fold when giving a medication.

Many programs use abbreviations that can be misunderstood—for example, 100 U can look like 1,000,
and the reader can easily add "units." Although a system may use DTO as an abbreviation for "deoderized
tincture of opium," the person using the computer
may think the abbreviation stands for "tincture of opium, diluted"; the outcome could be fatal if these drugs
are confused.

Some computers require the health care provider to
type in a patient's name to pull up his record; if the
name is misspelled, or if two patients have the same or
similar names, the wrong record may come up and
drugs may be ordered for the wrong patient. In addition, when checklists are used and a drug has to be selected from a long list of drugs, it's easy to check the
wrong drug, and a medication error might occur.

PREVENT IT

Medication error: Jacob, age 24, had been disabled with psychotic disease since age 20. After 6 months on the antipsychotic drug quetiapine (Seroquel), he began to function normally. He was holding down a job and living on his own, close to his family. The health care team was very pleased with his progress and at his 6-week review it was decided to continue the Seroquel and review his case in 2 months. The physician checked the new drug order system and clicked on Seroquel 400 mg/day with a refill in 4 weeks.

Two weeks after the session, Jacob was seen in the ED after a full psychotic episode. He was admitted to the psychiatric unit of the hospital for evaluation. His mother brought in his medications from his apartment, and it was discovered that he had been taking nefazodone (Serzone), an antidepressant, instead of Seroquel for the previous 2 weeks.

The physician checked with the pharmacy and the medication record and found an order for Serzone. Because this error couldn't have stemmed from handwriting misinterpretation, the physician went back to the ordering system to find the source of the problem. He discovered that Seroquel and Serzone were in alphabetical order on the list and that he had inadvertently clicked on the wrong drug. Because the dose could have been 400 mg/day for either drug, the mistake was overlooked.

Prevention: Like so many medication errors, patient education might have prevented this medication error. If Jacob had been instructed to look at his pills and question if they did not look the same as his previous pills or knew to check the drug name carefully when getting refills, he might have spotted the error. The prescriber, by his own admission, might have prevented the error if he was paying full attention to the computer screen when he selected the drug name. He stated that this system was so easy, he never really had to think, just point and click.

Although electronic and preprinted forms help alleviate some of the problems associated with handwriting misinterpretation and misheard doses and drug names, they introduce other potential sources of errors and, perhaps most dangerous, tend to lull people into a false sense of security—that all of the checks have been made and everything is safe, which results in less diligence. Even with computerized or preprinted and standardized forms, it's always important to check that the right patient is getting the right drug at the right dose by the right route at the right time.

✦ Proper care of drugs

Giving the right drug to the right patient includes giving a drug that has been stored under the right conditions. Some drugs come with specific storage directions—for example, refrigerate or protect from light. Some drugs tend to be relatively unstable compounds that could change if unprotected by special storage measures. With unit-dose medications, it may not be possible to know for sure if a drug was stored correctly before it arrived for administration. However, if a drug is known to require special storage, it should be checked for signs of improper storage. These signs include the formation of precipitates in the solutions, changes in color, or odd odors.

PREVENT IT

Medication error: Jamie Cribs, age 38, had been taking ganciclovir (Cytovene) every 12 hours for 7 days to treat cytomegalovirus retinitis. When the next dose arrived from the pharmacy, the nurse noticed particulate matter in the solution and thought that it appeared darker than previous doses. She tried shaking the bag, but the particles didn't dissolve. It was the weekend and the pharmacist wasn't on duty. The drugs for the weekend had been prepared earlier by the pharmacy and were stored on the unit. Believing that the patient had to have the drug, the nurse started the infusion and called the pharmacy supervisor at home to check on the drug. The supervisor told the nurse to stop the infusion immediately and that she would come in and prepare a new infusion.

Prevention: *Checking the other doses that had been prepared in advance revealed that these bags had been stored in the refrigerator on the unit. The pharmacist who had prepared the solutions noticed that they were stable for only 12 hours after being reconstituted; she felt that storing them in the refrigerator would prolong their stability through the weekend.*

However, ganciclovir shouldn't be stored in the refrigerator after being reconstituted. The pharmacist was new to this area of medicine and hadn't read all the instructions concerning the drug. The nurse, noting the particulate matter and the change in color of the drug, should have questioned the solution before infusing the drug.

Luckily, the patient didn't seem to have adverse effects, and this incident alerted the service that pharmacist coverage was needed throughout the weekend. A severe pharmacist shortage in the area had led to staff premixing solutions that were needed during the weekend. A careful review led to a posting of the drugs that can't be prepared ahead in this way.

Is it effective?

In some cases, although there's no apparent change in the drug and administering it to the patient may not cause immediate harm, the drug may no longer be effective, which may ultimately be harmful to the patient.

Nitroglycerin, a drug used for emergency relief of angina pain, is very unstable and must be stored away from light in a tightly closed bottle. Even with this precaution, this drug will still break down over time and become ineffective. Both staff and patients need to be aware of this fact so that they will be sure to check the expiration date and verify that the drug has been properly stored. However, the only way to really tell if nitroglycerin has become ineffective is when it fails to work. Tell patients to anticipate a tingling or fizzing under the tongue when nitroglycerin is placed there. If this doesn't occur, the drug is no longer active.

Aspirin is another drug that deteriorates with time. It's an over-the-counter (OTC) drug that patients might buy on sale and store for future use. In health care facilities, it's usually assumed that aspirin use is so high that nothing sits on the shelf very long. However, an old bottle can sometimes sit too long. Ineffective aspirin emits a vinegar-like odor that indicates that the drug is too old for therapeutic use; consumers should know that aspirin that smells vinegary shouldn't be used.

PREVENT IT

Medication error: *Jane Lasker, age 85, was prescribed sublingual nitroglycerin to relieve chest pain following what was believed to be an angina attack at a friend's funeral. She didn't need the tablets again until about 18 months later, when she suffered a severe angina attack with diaphoresis and chest and arm pain. She retrieved her bottle of nitroglycerin and followed the instructions to use a total of five tablets before going to the ED. After experiencing no relief, she went to the ED, where physicians confirmed that she was experiencing an angina attack. She obtained immediate relief from her chest pain after receiving a single nitroglycerin tablet sublingually. She was monitored for a short time and then released with a follow-up appointment with a cardiologist.*

Prevention: Following the medication instructions, the patient had left her nitroglycerin in the brown bottle that it came in and stored it in a drawer away from light. What she didn't follow was that the nitroglycerin should be replaced at least every 6 months. She thought that was a trick to make her buy more tablets and saw no reason to dispose of the unused drug. The nurse carefully reviewed the directions with the patient again, including the "fizzing" or "tingling" feeling under the tongue, and explained that her tablets were ineffective because the ingredients were no longer active. This error could have been prevented if the bottle had been clearly marked with an expiration date and the patient given written instructions to replace the bottle after a certain date.

Many patients have medicine cabinets full of drugs that have passed their expiration date, yet they continue to use these drugs to self-medicate. Some of these drugs could cause serious problems if used — the patient in the previous scenario could have suffered a serious myocardial infarction (MI) waiting for the nitroglycerin to work. In the hospital, it's a good idea to ask patients using sublingual nitroglycerin if they feel tingling or fizzing when the drug is under the tongue. This is a simple check of the drug's effectiveness.

Label it!

Drugs that require special storage should be clearly labeled with storage information and instructions. Many antibiotic suspensions need to be refrigerated; other drugs shouldn't be refrigerated. This information should be clearly stated on the label and reviewed with the patient, parents, or caregivers when the drug is dispensed for home use.

The patient who self-administers parenteral drugs, such as insulin or interferons, needs information on the proper storage of those drugs, many of which need to be refrigerated or stored in a cool place. Errors in drug storage at home can be prevented by careful and accurate patient education. The pharmacist, prescriber, and nurse should all reinforce this information. It's very important to make sure that the patient understands the information that's being given. Always ask the patient to repeat your instructions, and reinforce medication guidelines with written information.

Putting drugs in their proper place

Some storage problems that can lead to errors involve the placement of the drug on a shelf, on a counter, or even in a pocket. When you don't find a drug in its expected place — the drug bin, the patient's medication drawer — carefully check the label before using the drug. Medication errors have occurred when drugs are left on a table or the wrong vial is picked up to prepare a syringe. An error can also occur when one syringe of medication is drawn up and accidentally picked up and used while another drug is being prepared because it wasn't properly labeled. These errors can be prevented by always taking the time to check the name of the drug against the medication administration record each time you handle it, even if you think you know exactly what it is.

PREVENT IT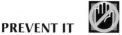

Medication error: A very busy, understaffed, skilled nursing care unit was overcrowded with 38 patients — two beds were in the hallway because all rooms were filled. The nurse assigned to dispense the medications for all the patients knew that many patients had glaucoma and were receiving eye drops each morning. Because many patients were on the same drug, the nurse kept the bottle in her uniform pocket and used the same bottle for everyone who needed the drug. This process helped her finish dispensing the morning medications in time to give the noon medications.

The same nurse was also responsible for performing stool quaiac testing that day. As the morning progressed, she became increasingly overwhelmed with the busy pace. The nurse put the quaiac testing solution in one pocket and the glaucoma medicine in the other.

At some point during the morning, a patient complained of eye pain after receiving the eye drops. The nurse knew that the patient was a complainer and was not concerned. When the next patient also complained, the nurse checked the bottle and realized that she had mistakenly switched the two solutions: she was using the quaiac testing solution as eye drops. Luckily, no one was seriously harmed.

Prevention: In clinical practice, shortcuts are sometimes used to survive the day. Although the nurse knew that the same bottle shouldn't be used to administer eye drops to different patients because of the risk of cross-contamination, she used this method to save time. Also, other nurses on this floor carried the quaiac testing solution in a pocket because policy required testing all stools. Having the solution always on hand saved time going to a central location when a test was needed. The white, plastic bottles of the two solutions looked similar, and it was easy to see how they were confused. The bottles should have never been stored in a pocket and pulled out when needed. The nurse assumed that she knew what she was administering because she had put the drug in her pocket and took it out only when eye drops were indicated.

Improper storage—the nurse's uniform pocket—led to this potentially serious error. Always check the label just before administering a drug. If the nurse in this case would have read the label, the error would have been prevented and the nurse may have realized the potential for further error and removed the drug from her pocket.

In some situations, drugs are left where patients or visitors have access to them. Topical drugs, such as topical steroids or antibiotics, may be left on a bedside stand for application when needed or they may be unconsciously left behind in the patient's room. These drugs should be carefully labeled and placed out of sight when not in use. Patients or visitors may inadvertently pick up these drugs and use or discard them, either of which could cause problems.

PREVENT IT

Medication error: *Mr. Davenport, a hospital patient, frantically rang his call bell and told the nurse that something was wrong with his wife. The nurse rushed to the room and found Mrs. Davenport slumped in the chair looking pale and complaining of a severe headache and dizziness. Her pulse was rapid and her blood pressure was very low.*

The nurse called the emergency response team, and Mrs. Davenport was taken to the ED for evaluation. The staff had to clean a sticky white paste off of the patient's arms and hands to apply monitoring electrodes and start an I.V. line. In a short period, her blood pressure returned to normal, her color improved, and she reported that her headache had gone away. All the tests done on Mrs. Davenport were within normal limits and she was discharged.

When visiting her husband the next day, Mrs. Davenport talked with the nursing staff about her strange and sudden illness. They discussed what she may have eaten and her activities that day. The only unusual thing that she could remember was using the creme that was on her husband's bedside stand. She said that her skin was very dry and she felt that creme used in a hospital would be good for her skin. She had picked up the creme from the bedside stand and applied it generously to her arms and hands.

Mr. Davenport was recovering from an acute MI and was receiving nitroglycerin paste three times daily. The crème that Mrs. Davenport had generously applied to her arms and hands was the nitroglycerin paste that the nurse had mistakenly left on the bedside stand. The signs and symptoms that Mrs. Davenport experienced were related to the effects of the very high dose of nitroglycerin.

Prevention: *This problem could have been prevented if the patient's medications had been properly stored and the patient's wife hadn't had the availability of the drug. Many reports describe patients or their families mistaking nitroglycerin paste for toothpaste, hair gel, or body creme. Other reports have involved patients mistaking glue for contact lens solutions or antibiotic eye medication; the resultant damage to the eye can be very traumatic.*

Reports about mix-ups like these are filed only after adverse effects have occurred. Drugs involved with such confusion need clear and obvious labeling, and patients being discharged with these drugs need strong reinforcement about their proper storage. Patients should also be taught to always check the label just before using these products.

Keep out of reach

Tragic medication errors have occurred when drugs weren't properly stored out of the reach of children. It's good policy to tell patients taking medication at home — prescription, OTC, or herbal — to keep it away from children. The adult dose for many drugs can be toxic, or even fatal, to small children. Children are very curious and like to imitate adults. If they see adults taking medication, they may also want to do so. The potential problems associated with children taking adult medications led to the development of childproof packaging. However, anyone with small children knows that these packages often prove more difficult for adults to open than children. Older adults with arthritis or weakness may remove the medication from the childproof package after they've opened it because they have difficulty reopening the packages. Some people keep their medications in plain sight, often not in their original containers, as a reminder to take the drugs. Such practices can have tragic results.

PREVENT IT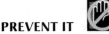

Medication error: *Lisa Little, age 28, suffered a miscarriage. She lost a great deal of blood during the miscarriage and underwent a dilation and curettage to control the bleeding. On her 6-week follow-up visit, she was found to have recovered physically from the event, but was still depressed over her loss. Her hematocrit was 31, and she admitted feeling tired and weak. She was offered emotional support and given a supply of ferrous sulfate tablets, with instructions to take one tablet three times per day.*

At home, she transferred the pills to a decorative bottle that had once held vitamins and left it on her table as a reminder to take the tablets. The next day, she discovered her 2-year-old daughter eating the tablets and punished her for getting into them. About 1 hour later, the toddler complained of a really bad "tummy ache" and started vomiting. The child then became lethargic. Ms. Little called the pediatrician, who told her take the child immediately to the ED and to take the remaining tablets with her.

The toddler was found to have a weak, rapid pulse (156 beats/minute); rapid, shallow respirations (32 breaths/minute); and low blood pressure (60/42 mm Hg). When a diagnosis of acute iron toxicity was made, Ms. Little became distraught. She said she had no idea that iron could be dangerous because it can be bought OTC in so many preparations. She hadn't read the written information given to her because it was "just iron."

The first priority was to support and detoxify the child. In cases of acute iron poisoning, the patient should be induced to vomit and given eggs and milk to bind the iron and prevent absorption. The patient may undergo gastric lavage, using a 1% sodium bicarbonate solution; this procedure is safe for the first hour after ingestion. After that time, there's an increased risk of gastric erosion caused by the corrosive iron, making lavage dangerous. Because the toddler was well beyond the first hour of iron ingestion, supportive measures to deal with shock, dehydration, and GI damage were necessary. In addition, an iron-chelating agent, such as deferoxamine mesylate, was used. Sadly, the toddler didn't recover.

Prevention: *Most people don't take OTC drugs seriously; many don't even read the labels—all the more reason to stress the importance of reading labels and following the directions that come with OTC drugs. This tragedy could have been avoided had Ms. Little received this type of instruction— not just written information—when she was instructed to take iron. The drug also shouldn't have been stored in an attractive bottle in full reach of a child. This was clearly the wrong drug for the wrong person.*

Special preparation

Some drugs require special preparation before they're given. For example, the sedative/hypnotic paraldehyde can be given rectally or orally to calm severely agitated patients or those with delirium tremens. Before it's given, this drug must be diluted in oil for retention enemas or in milk or iced fruit juice for oral use. The drug shouldn't come in contact with plastic because it reacts with and destroys the plastic. Also, it shouldn't be exposed to the air and open containers must be discarded; it shouldn't be stored in warm areas or in sunlight. If the solution appears to be brown or smells of vinegar, it's no longer safe to use and should be discarded. When prepared properly, the drug should be given immediately. Paraldehyde is a prime example of a drug that requires proper preparation; the storage, dilution, and administration requirements are complex. However, it's also a good example of how important it is to review dilution and preparation requirements before giving a drug.

PREVENT IT

Medication error: Todd Leyton, a 58-year-old chronic alcoholic, was admitted to the ED with acute delirium tremens on an extremely busy Saturday night. Because the patient had visited the ED in the past, the staff was familiar with his behavior and responses. Paraldehyde was ordered to calm him and help him sleep. The nurse mixed the paraldehyde with cold orange juice, but was called to help another nurse before she could administer the drug. When she returned a few minutes later, Todd was even more agitated, accusing the nurse of trying to kill him. Not knowing the problems with paraldehyde and plastic, the nurse had mixed the drug in a plastic cup using a plastic spoon. The cup and spoon were dissolving on the bedside stand.

Prevention: It's always a good idea to check for special instructions when diluting a drug. If a drug is used frequently in an area, as paraldehyde is in the ED, a notice should be posted regarding diluting instructions and special precautions. If you aren't familiar with a drug and need to dilute it, always investigate how it should be properly diluted or prepared.

Cutting and crushing medications

Drug administration can be a challenge when patients, because of age or medical condition, find it difficult to swallow pills whole. In the past, it was standard nursing procedure to cut or crush medications to make them easier to swallow. Mixing crushed tablets or emptying capsules into applesauce, pudding, or ice cream was common; in some cases, crushed medications were also delivered through nasogastric or feeding tubes. Medication carts commonly are equipped with mortars and pestles for crushing pills. Unit-dose packages can be opened and the tablets cut or crushed, or the capsules opened and the contents spilled into liquid or soft food. This common practice, however, has become a dangerous practice.

Modern technology has led to the development of drug delivery systems that permit a more consistent therapeutic serum level of some drugs that are administered only once or twice a day instead of around the clock. Many of these systems are designed to gradually release the drug from an insoluble shell at a controlled rate. Cutting, crushing, or chewing these medications alters the delivery system and destroys their slow-release properties. When swallowing the crushed substance, the patient receives an overlarge — potentially toxic — initial dose of the drug and then subtherapeutic levels of the drug throughout the rest of the day.

This preparation error can be avoided with proper education. Patients who are prescribed drugs that can't be cut, crushed, or chewed need to receive written guidelines about the dangers of doing so. Nursing units should post a list of the drugs that can't be cut, crushed, or chewed. In some long-term care facilities, crushing the patients' medications has been the routine. "We've always done it that way" isn't an acceptable reason for crushing all pills now — this practice is no longer safe.

PREVENT IT

Medication error: Carl Root, a recently retired engineer, had been taken nifedipine (Procardia XL) 60 mg/day orally to control his hypertension. At his last office visit, the nurse noted that his blood pressure was quite low: 106/60 mm Hg. He was given a new prescription for nifedipine, 30 mg/day, and asked to record his blood pressure at home and return in 6 weeks. During that time, his wife called the office to report that Mr. Root had been breaking out in a sweat, becoming jittery and dizzy, complaining of being nauseated, and having a tingling sensation in his arms and legs every day about a half hour after taking his new dose of medication. Within a few hours, the symptoms pass and he's fine for the rest of the day. She was concerned that the dose might not be right.

When Mr. Root came into the office that afternoon, his blood pressure was 180/102 mm Hg. He explained that he had just filled his prescription for the 60 mg Procardia XL before the dose was changed. He's on a fixed income and his insurance won't pay for another refill of the same drug at this time. Seeing that the new dose was half of the old dose, he had purchased a pill cutter at the pharmacy and cut all of his pills in half so that he wouldn't waste money and would still get 30 mg of the drug.

This was an understandable but misguided plan. By cutting the tablets and taking only half, Mr. Root had destroyed the sustained-release properties of the drug. He got the full effects of the 30-mg dose within a half hour of taking the drug; the dizziness and other events were predictable adverse effects of the drug. The drug has a half-life of 2 to 5 hours. Later in the day, the symptoms passed.

Prevention: Many patients cut tablets in half or empty capsules to help them swallow the medication. Some patients are even encouraged to cut the tablets to save money when a large dose of the drug is actually cheaper than many small doses. However, it's always important to check whether the *drug can be cut, crushed, or chewed. Generally, if a drug is "sustained release" or "extended release," it probably shouldn't be manipulated.*

Patients should receive written information and have the instructions explained to them before they start using "untouchable" drugs in the home. Although things may have "always been done this way" in various nursing facilities, information should be posted regarding drugs that can't be cut, crushed, or chewed today. Unit-dose medications should include warnings from the pharmacy. This type or error can be prevented with good education. (See Drugs that can't be cut.*)*

Forgetting the rules

Improper preparation can also occur when the use of a medication becomes routine and preparation details are forgotten. Some drug solutions need to be shaken well before each use. Cefdinir (Omnicef) is an antibiotic available in an oral suspension that must be stored at room temperature and shaken well before each use to ensure that the drug is properly suspended in the solution. The patient may follow the instruction to shake the suspension when he's taking the first dose; however, by day four or five, he may just pour the dose from the bottle. Much of the drug will have precipitated to the bottom of the bottle, and the patient won't receive the intended dose. Such drugs should come with clear instructions on the label explaining the need to shake the drug well before every use. It may also be helpful to demonstrate how to shake a bottle well.

There are other drugs that require proper preparation. An insulin pen is a convenient delivery device that allows the busy patient to administer insulin inconspicuously during the day. A cartridge of insulin is inserted into the pen, and the pen must be rotated 15

Drugs that can't be cut

Tablets and capsules that can't be cut, crushed, or chewed are listed below. If you work in an area that uses these drugs regularly, copy the list and post it in your work area as a reminder about the proper preparation of these drugs.

TABLETS/CAPSULES THAT CAN'T BE CUT, CRUSHED, OR CHEWED

✦ acitretin (Soriatane)
✦ aminophylline (Phyllocontin)
✦ aspirin (ZORprin, Bayer Extended Release)
✦ benzonatate (Tessalon, Benzonatate Softgels)
✦ bisacodyl (Ducolax)
✦ budesonide (Entocort)
✦ carbamazepine (Tegretol-XR)
✦ cefaclor (Ceclor CD)
✦ chloral hydrate (Aquachloral Supprettes)
✦ chlorpheniramine (Chlor-Trimeton Allergy)
✦ chlorpromazine (Thorazine Spansule)
✦ clarithromycin (Biaxin)
✦ colestipol (Colestid)
✦ dexchlorpheniramine (Polaramine Repetabs)
✦ dextroamphetamine (Dexedrine Spansule)
✦ diethylpropion (Tenuate)
✦ diflunisal (Dolobid)
✦ diltiazem (Dilacor-XR)
✦ dirithromycin (Dynabac)
✦ disopyramide (Norpace CR)
✦ divalproex (Depakote)
✦ esomeprazole (Nexium)
✦ etretinate (Tegison)
✦ felodipine (Plendil)
✦ fluphenazine (Prolixin)
✦ gatifloxacin (Tequin)
✦ isosorbide (SR and ER preparation)
✦ isotretinoin (Accutane)

(continued)

Drugs that can't be cut *(continued)*

✦ lansoprazole (Prevacid)
✦ meprobamate (Equanil)
✦ mesalamine (Asacol)
✦ methylphenidate (Ritalin SR, Concerta)
✦ metoprolol (Toprol-XL)
✦ morphine (MS Contin, Oramorph SR)
✦ nifedipine (Adalat CC, Procardia XL)
✦ nisoldipine (Sular)
✦ nitroglycerin (Nitroglyn, Nitrong, Nitro-time)
✦ norfloxacin (Noroxin)
✦ omeprazole (Prilosec)
✦ ondansetron (Zofran)
✦ orphenadrine (Norflex)
✦ oxtriphylline (Choledyl SA)
✦ oxycodone (OxyContin)
✦ pancrelipase (Cotazym, Ku-Zyme)
✦ pancreatin (Creon Capsules, Donnazyme)
✦ pantoprazole (Protonix)
✦ paroxetine CR (Paxil CR)
✦ pentoxifylline (Trental)
✦ potassium chloride (Kaon-Cl, Slow-K, Ten-K, K-Dur)
✦ procainamide (Procanbid, Pronestyl-SR)
✦ prochlorperazine (Compazine)
✦ quinidine (Quinidex Extentabs, Quinabin, Quinaglute Dura-Tabs)
✦ rabeprazole (Aciphex)
✦ sulfasalazine (Azulfidine EN-Tabs)
✦ tamsulosin (Flomax)
✦ temozolomide (Temodal)
✦ theophylline (Theodur)
✦ topiramate (Topamax)
✦ tripelennamine (PBZ-SR)
✦ typhoid vaccine, oral (Vivotif Berna)
✦ valproic acid (Depakote)
✦ verapamil (Calan SR, Isoptin SR)

to 20 times to properly suspend the insulin before it's injected. When the patient first uses an insulin pen, he's educated about drug preparation before he injects the insulin. The patient who uses other injections or inhalers also needs to be taught about drug preparation before becoming responsible for his drug regimen.

Commonly, the patient is asked to repeat the process for the nurse or teacher when first learning how to use the device. After a patient has been using the device for some time, however, the ability to use the device is assumed and the patient's technique isn't checked. As with all habits, the patient forgets details over time or picks up and incorporates an error into the routine.

When the proper preparation of a drug is essential to obtain its therapeutic effect, it's important to reinforce the details of drug preparation each time the patient is seen. Don't just ask the patient if he's preparing the drug correctly; ask him to show you how he prepares the drug. If this isn't practical because of time constraints, it would be advisable to make a note in the patient's chart to check preparation and technique at least once a year for chronically used drugs.

PREVENT IT

Medication error: James Wells, a 52-year-old financial consultant who travels extensively, has diabetes and eats most of his meals away from home. He had difficulty carrying and using his insulin before meals until the introduction of the insulin pen. This system allowed him to easily administer his insulin in many settings and situations. Mr. Wells was very excited when he got the new device and attended an educational session with the diabetic nurse educator, which included discussion of the important preparation step — rotating the *pen 15 to 20 times to ensure that the insulin is adequately suspended.*

Over the past 2 months, Mr. Wells had been having an increasing number of hypoglycemic episodes, but his travel schedule had made it impossible for him to see his health care provider. During an important dinner conference, Mr. Wells became dizzy, confused, and shaky, and he passed out for a few seconds. He was rushed to the area ED by the convention center emergency response team. During transit, a fingerstick glucose test showed that his blood sugar was a very low 36 mg/dl. The team started an I.V. line with dextrose 5% in water and gave him some oral glucose tablets. On arrival, his fingerstick blood sugar was 95 mg/dl and they decided to continue to treat him with oral glucose tablets.

In a short time, his blood sugar returned to a normal range and he was able to discuss the situation with the nurse. Mr. Wells denied changes in his diet, exercise, or medications. He said that he had given himself his insulin after checking the date on the new cartridge to make sure it hadn't expired. Although he admitted that he doesn't rotate injection sites very often because it's inconvenient with his hectic schedule, he didn't think that would have caused this problem.

On returning home, Mr. Wells met with the diabetic nurse for a refresher program at his physician's insistence. The nurse found that he had a very good understanding of his disease, exercise, diet, and insulin therapy. However, when asked to demonstrate how he administered his insulin, Mr. Wells took the pen, tilted it twice, and injected the insulin. He had completely forgotten that the pen needed to be rotated 15 to 20 times before injection; Mr. Wells was probably not getting the expected dose of insulin when he injected the drug.

Prevention: *Careful and repetitive patient teaching could have prevented this medication error. Although Mr. Wells' hectic travel and work schedule made return visits to his health care provider less frequent, those visits should have included a review of the preparation and administration of his medication. It's important to ask the patient to demonstrate* *how he administers the drug, whether it's by injection, in-haler, or dermal patch. By watching the patient demonstrate the process, the nurse can evaluate how instructions were in-terpreted and how the patient's understanding of the proce-dure may have changed over time.*

IT'S A FACT

Studies of the effectiveness of insulin pens have shown a vari-ation from 5% to 224% of the expected concentration of in-sulin when the insulin isn't suspended properly before ad-ministration. The variations typically occur when the car-tridge is new.

✦ Using common sense

A last check in determining if you're giving the right drug is to check to see if that drug makes sense for the patient. For beginning nurses or for nurses new to a particular field of nursing, this may mean spending time looking up a drug's actions, indications, con-traindications, and possible adverse effects before ad-ministering it. If it's an emergency or high-pressure sit-uation where there isn't time to look up a drug, it may mean asking someone familiar with the drug to ex-plain its use or to be responsible for its administration.

You're responsible for your actions. Don't rely on other people's judgment when it comes to administer-ing medications. Ask the prescriber for the indication for which the drug is being given. Your questions should become standard practice: "Please give me the generic name, brand name, and indication." If a busy prescriber doesn't have the patience to explain all parts of a drug order, it isn't unreasonable to refuse to administer the drug. Instructions such as "That's what was ordered, so give it," "This is a special situation," or "This is a particular drug protocol" are unacceptable. If you don't understand why a drug is being given to a patient, if it doesn't make sense to you, or if it seems wrong, check it out and don't give the drug until you receive a reasonable explanation.

PREVENT IT

Medication error: Two young men were sharing a room on a busy surgical unit. One patient was recovering from a complicated appendectomy and peritonitis, but was otherwise healthy. The other patient had undergone surgery for Hodgkin's disease and was being started on chlorambucil (Leukeran) as the first course of chemotherapy. Both men had arrived the same day and had been given a workup by a fourth-year medical student. The student was overwhelmed by the workload and was quite rushed as he wrote up the patients' charts and their orders. When the oncologist gave the order for chlorambucil, the student inadvertently wrote it on the wrong patient's chart.

The man recovering from the appendectomy was given several days of chemotherapy before his blood work showed a severe bone marrow depression; this led to the discovery that he was getting an antineoplastic drug. The oncologist had never cosigned the student's order because he never saw it; the nurse caring for the patient and the pharmacist dispensing the drug failed to check the patient's diagnosis before giving or dispensing the drug, and the patient failed to ask about the medication he was receiving.

Prevention: Several errors occurred in this situation. Ultimately, the patient received the wrong drug. Before administering a drug to a patient, it's important, while checking for identification, allergies, and use of other drugs, to know the patient's diagnosis. Make sure that the drug you're giving

*makes sense for the diagnosis or patient history. The patient
in the previous example had an infection and an appendectomy. If the nurse had known that diagnosis, it should have
triggered questions about why this patient was being given an
antineoplastic agent.*

Alternative uses for medications

Despite knowing the patient's diagnosis and the approved indications for a particular drug, sometimes
questions still may arise when a drug is ordered. Many
drugs are used for indications that aren't on the "approved indications" list; these uses are referred to as
"off-label" uses. Sometimes, these uses can be found in
the "unlabeled uses" section of a drug monograph.
These uses may also be particular to a certain area or
prescriber. Usually, off-label uses are commonly applied to pediatric patients because drug research on
this age group is limited, preventing pediatric patients
from being included on the approved list. In addition,
many of the drugs used for psychiatric disorders aren't
indicated for the diagnosis of a particular patient for
whom it has been ordered, but experience with the
drug has led to its use for that disorder.

Gabapentin (Neurontin) is approved for the treatment of specific seizure disorders. However, the drug
has also been found to be effective in treating patients
who are depressed, anxious, or paranoid, as well as
those suffering from other psychiatric disorders. Physicians have tried using this drug, commonly combined
with other drugs, to achieve a specific effect. If gabapentin is ordered for a patient with a diagnosis of depression and the nurse checks the drug's approved indications, she won't find depression. The nurse now
has to decide whether it's appropriate to give the drug.
If it's accepted medical practice in the area to use the

drug for unlisted indications, it may be sufficient to discuss this with the prescriber or the nursing supervisor for reassurance that this is the right drug for the patient. If you work in a field where off-label drug use is common, it may be a good idea to check into the policies that cover administration of these drugs. Another important factor to consider when giving a patient a drug for an off-label use is to inform the patient what the drug is being given for; he should know the generic and brand names of his drugs, dosages, and indications. This is especially important with off-label uses because other health care providers, who may see the patient on consult or in an emergency situation, may not know why the patient is receiving that drug, and problems with diagnosis or treatment could arise. Generally, the standard drug printout that's given to the patient at the pharmacy won't explain off-label uses. Also, pharmacists commonly aren't able to alter these standard drug sheets and may not have the time to write in other indications. A customized, written teaching sheet about the drug, including the specific indication for the patient, is important for the prescriber to provide to prevent future problems with off-label uses of drugs.

PREVENT IT

Medication error: *A woman with a chronic neurogenic pain syndrome was prescribed amitriptyline (Elavil), an antidepressant, as adjunctive therapy. Her physician didn't discuss the drug with her; he just told her that it was something else she should try.*

When the woman had the prescription filled at her local pharmacy, the pharmacist told her that he had included instructions for taking the antidepressant. The woman was startled to discover that the physician had ordered an antide-

---

✦

Drug safety checklist

Use this quick checklist to help prevent medication errors.

RIGHT DRUG

☐ Check the generic name, brand name, and intended indication of the drug twice—when preparing the drug and just before administering it.

☐ Check that the drug makes sense for the patient.

☐ Check that the drug has been stored properly.

☐ Check that the drug has been prepared properly.

---

pressant and assumed he had decided the pain was all in her mind. She refused the medication and informed the physician that she was upset and was switching to a new physician. At this point, the explanation that amitriptyline has an unlabeled use for adjunctive therapy in the treatment of various pain syndromes wasn't sufficient to undo the stress and irritation that the woman had experienced.

***Prevention:** Lack of communication led to this medication problem. If the physician had discussed the drug with the patient and explained its uses or if he had noted the intended indication on the prescription, this problem might have been avoided. By not informing the patient about the drug and its intended use, the physician placed the patient in a precarious situation. Other health care providers seeing this patient would note the drug and most likely assume that it was being given as an antidepressant—depression being the approved indication. The patient's evaluation and treatment would be changed because of this assumption. Although this drug was the right drug for this patient, its use needed explanation to prevent an error.*

✦ Replay: The second right

The second right in the common-sense approach to preventing medication errors is to make sure that the drug you're going to give is the right drug. This involves verifying many different factors. It may sound complicated, but going through a quick checklist in your mind before administering a drug can prevent the medication errors that result from giving the wrong drug to the patient. (See *Drug safety checklist*, page 153.)

The right dose

The third "right" to consider before administering a drug is whether the dose you're about to give is the "right dose." This means ensuring that it has been interpreted and calculated correctly and that individual variations that could require alteration in the correct therapeutic dose, such as the patient's weight, have been taken into account.

✦ Making the correct interpretation

Problems involving interpreting the ordered dose of a drug are similar to those encountered when trying to interpret the ordered type of drug.

Problems with the writing

Poor handwriting, poor communication skills, and distractions can result in a misinterpretation of the intended dose. It's always a good idea to check it in a current nursing drug guide, especially if you aren't familiar with the particular drug or its specific use. Looking up the recommended dosage can alert you to a misinterpreted order or — if the ordered dose is wrong — an inaccurate order.

PREVENT IT

> ***Medication error:*** *A resident was asked to evaluate a post-partum woman with a sexually transmitted disease. He wrote the following order: penicillin G.5 million units q4h. To the nurse, the G looked like a 6 and, because it was so close to the .5, it appeared that the order was 6.5 million units. The student nurse assigned to that patient was required to look up her patient's drugs before administering them and noticed that this was a very high dose for penicillin. She alerted her instructor, who concurred. They called the physician, who verified the error and corrected the order. Everyone agreed that the resident's sloppy handwriting was hard to decipher.*
>
> ***Prevention:*** *A prescriber's illegible handwriting should alert the person reading the order that interpretation of the drug dose may be difficult. The best way to prevent errors involving misinterpretation of written orders is to always check it out. It's easy for the brain to be fooled when something looks familiar. We often leap ahead and assume that what's written is correct because it looks correct. Remember, "When in doubt, check it out."*

Problems with the reading

Another frequently reported error is the misreading of the end of a drug name as the first number in an order. When the drug name and the dosage are written very closely together, the human eye can interpret these as a name and a distinct number.

PREVENT IT

> ***Medication error:*** *A patient was discharged following a myocardial infarction with the following order: Inderal 40 mg P.O. The order was interpreted at the pharmacy as Inderal*

140 mg; the "l" at the end of the word Inderal seen as a "1." Although the pharmacist knew the drug name well and read it correctly, he mistakenly saw 140 as the dose. He thought that was a rather high dose on which to start the patient and questioned the physician. Although the physician was sure he hadn't ordered that dose, when the pharmacist checked the order, he still read it as Inderal 140 mg. The physician corrected the order to 40 mg. Later, the pharmacist and his supervisor discussed the problem. When the supervisor looked at the order, she saw it as Inderal 40, and they were able to sort out the confusion. When the problem was obvious, the pharmacist couldn't believe he had read the dose in such a different way.

*   **Prevention:** *Drug names that end in "i" or "l" should be red flags to anyone reading orders because they're known to cause confusion. It's also a good idea to double-check an order that has run-on words or numbers. If the handwriting has the drug name, dosage and, perhaps, route run together, it should signal the potential for misinterpretation. When in doubt, check it out.*

Problems with the decimal point

Misinterpretation of an ordered dose is more likely to happen when it's unclear where the decimal point is placed. It's important to always use a zero before a decimal point when the ordered dose is less than one measurement unit. For example, in the error discussed earlier in the chapter, ".5 million units" should have read "0.5 million units." That would have alerted the nurse transcribing the order to a different meaning; 6.05 million units would have been very inappropriate and the nurse probably would have detected the transcription error immediately. Without a zero preceding it, the decimal point can easily be lost in the reading or transcription of the order. A small decimal is easy to overlook when you're busy, distracted, or unfamiliar with a particular drug.

IT'S A FACT

In April 2001, the Washington Post reported a tragic medication error involving the decimal point. A physician ordered morphine .5 mg I.V. q2h as needed for postoperative pain in a 9-month-old girl. The unit secretary transcribing the order didn't see the decimal point, and wrote the order for 5 mg intravenously (I.V.). The nurse caring for the child had been floated to the pediatric unit from an adult intensive care unit (ICU) because of a staffing shortage. The dose of 5 mg didn't seem odd to her, and she checked the medication record before giving the drug. She gave the initial 5 mg and repeated the dose in 2 hours. About 4 hours later, the baby suffered a cardiac arrest and died.

It's impossible to control staffing shortages in today's market and every effort has to be made to ensure patient safety. Stress the mandatory use of the zero preceding a decimal point if the dose ordered is less than one whole unit of measure. This error has been reported repeatedly in the literature. Although the use of computerized systems doesn't guarantee that this error won't occur, some systems routinely use a decimal point for drug dosages. It remains the responsibility of the person administering the drug to ensure that the patient is receiving the right dose.

Problems with the zero
Conversely, adding a zero *after* a decimal point when the dose needed is a whole number can cause confusion and misinterpretation of the order as well. If the decimal point is missed, the misinterpretation could re-

sult in a dose that's 10 to 100 times the intended dose. If an order seems to be beyond the norm, always question it. Sometimes, reviewing the medication record—even a computer-generated printout—isn't enough. Some computer systems automatically add zeros after a decimal point. Although this serves the computer system well, it can cause confusion. Review the original order or check directly with the prescriber. When in doubt, check it out.

PREVENT IT

Medication error: A patient with a long-standing history of phlebitis had taken warfarin (Coumadin) in the past to prevent thrombi formation. When she was seen for what appeared to be a new episode of phlebitis, her physician decided to start her immediately on 1 mg of warfarin. When he wrote the order, he used a prepared "DAW" (dispense as written) prescription form that was given to him by the company that makes Coumadin. He wrote: 1.0 mg Coumadin P.O. with a follow-up prothrombin time in 2 days. The form had lines printed on it, which obscured the decimal point in the order, and the pharmacist read the order as 10 mg.

The prescription was filled with 10 mg of the drug, and when the patient returned to the clinic to have her prothrombin time evaluated after 2 days, it was 38 seconds with a control of 12, which is very high. The physician was called and he instructed her to stop taking the Coumadin. The clinic staff gave her vitamin K as the antidote for warfarin overdose. The physician, very upset, asked the pharmacy for an explanation. The original order was faxed over to him, and he agreed that the decimal point was lost on the line and that the order did appear to read 10 mg.

Prevention: This problem could have been prevented if the prescriber hadn't written a zero after a dose that was a whole number. Every effort should be made to keep the dos-

ing information as simple and straightforward as possible. Many computer systems add or require a decimal point and zeros to fit into an order template. This can cause problems when orders are read or interpreted. Again, if an order seems outside the norm, be sure to question it.

Problems with abbreviations

There are many generally accepted abbreviations used in health care. However, problems can occur when abbreviations are used that aren't standard or are misinterpreted. In recent years, there have been several reports of errors involving the use of "U" for units—a measurement used in drugs, such as insulin and heparin. The "U" can be misread as a zero or a four if a person's handwriting is less than perfect or hurried, leading to a potential drug overdose.

IT'S A FACT

In late 2001, The American Diabetes Association delivered a policy statement calling for an end to the use of "U" in correspondence or literature. It suggested that all prescribers write out the word "unit" to clarify the meaning and prevent future errors.

There have also been many mix-ups when "IU"—an abbreviation for international units—has been misread as "I.V.," leading to serious dosage and administration route errors in some patients. Reports of errors have also been noted when "cc" (cubic centimeters) has been misread as "u" (unit). This can be a serious issue if a drug comes in units and can be administered in cubic centimeters.

PREVENT IT

Medication error: A resident wrote an order for 4U of regular insulin to be given 30 minutes before breakfast. The nurse who was filling in for the unit secretary glanced at the order and transcribed it as 40 units. She knew that insulin comes in units and assumed that it would be units. She misread the resident's handwriting as 40, not 4U, filling in the "units" herself. The patient received 40 units of insulin the next morning and, when she refused to eat breakfast, became severely hypoglycemic and required treatment. When the nurse checked back on the order sheet, she immediately realized what had happened when she saw the resident's handwriting.

Prevention: Following the lead of the American Diabetes Association, it would be wise to always spell out the word "units." This error would have been avoided if the "U" had been written out as "units." Although this may initially be a difficult habit to get into if you have been in clinical practice for some time, it could prevent many medication errors.

Problems with "sound-alike" dosages

It's important to be aware of reported confusion with sound-alike doses, such as:

- ✦ thirteen and thirty
- ✦ fourteen and forty
- ✦ fifteen and fifty
- ✦ sixteen and sixty
- ✦ seventeen and seventy
- ✦ eighteen and eighty
- ✦ nineteen and ninety.

If a verbal order is given for any of these units for any drug, always repeat that order; for example, by saying "one-five" or "five-zero." This will clarify the order and alert all parties that an error is possible.

PREVENT IT

Medication error: A 48-year-old man with severe hypertension was admitted to the emergency department (ED) from his physician's office. The physician phoned in an order for 15 mg hydralazine I.V. every 2 hours to be started immediately. The nurse taking the order thought that the physician said 50 mg hydralazine. She went to the floor stock, found 20 mg vials of hydralazine, drew up 2½ vials, and administered them to the patient. Within a few minutes, the patient's blood pressure dropped to a dangerously low level, and supportive measures were begun. When reviewing the incident, the nurse looked up the drug in a drug guide and found that 50 mg is a very high dose for this drug. When the physician arrived at the ED, he looked at the order and realized the mistake.

Prevention: This mistake could have been avoided if the nurse had asked the prescriber to verify the order: "Do you mean 50, 5-0 mg?" This would have alerted the prescriber to the misunderstanding. Remember to verify any number that could be confusing.

Problems with numbers

There are situations in which a prescriber orders one unit of a drug—for example, one tablet or one capsule. Sometimes this happens because the prescriber is trying to keep things simple for the patient; other times, the prescriber is just accustomed to ordering a drug that way and may have forgotten the dose contained in one unit. This can become a problem when a drug comes out in a new preparation, which happens frequently, or when a person moves to a new area where drugs are available in different preparations.

Never accept an order for a specific number of tablets, capsules, or vials. Always request that the prescriber give the correct dose. This provides another check in the system. If the dose ordered isn't available as one tablet or capsule, then verify the order—it may be that the wrong drug is being used or the wrong dose was calculated.

PREVENT IT

Medication error: A 78-year-old patient in a nursing home had been unable to sleep, and the nurse called the physician to prescribe a sleeping pill. The physician stated that the nurse should give the patient "one chloral hydrate capsule at bedtime" if the problem persisted. That evening, the patient complained that she was unable to sleep; the nurse checked the floor stock and found 500-mg capsules of chloral hydrate. Checking the order, she gave one capsule to the patient. Later, thinking about how small the elderly patient was, the nurse looked up the drug to see if it came in more than one size capsule. She discovered that it was also available in a 250-mg capsule. She called the physician the next day to check on the dose. He told the nurse that he assumed the nursing home would stock the smaller dose of the capsule, and the order was rewritten to include the strength and number of capsules.

Prevention: No one can keep up with all available forms of every drug. If an order is written that doesn't specify a precise dose of the drug, verify that order. If a precise dose isn't written, the possibilities of error are wide-ranging. If you feel uncomfortable confronting a prescriber for the precise information, look it up beforehand so you can discuss the range of possibilities. Don't give a tablet or capsule or use an ampule without direct information about what's intended for the patient.

Factors in verifying drug dosages

Consider these points when verifying a specific drug dose for the patient:

✦ Weight: Because recommended dosages typically are based on a 150-lb (68-kg) adult male, the patient who's much lighter or much heavier may need a dose adjustment to get the intended therapeutic effect from the drug.

✦ Age: Patients at the extremes of the age spectrum — children and older adults — commonly require dosage adjustments based on the functional level of their livers and kidneys and the responsiveness of their other organs. Also, always ask women of childbearing age about the possibility of pregnancy before you give them a drug.

✦ Physical parameters related to the disease state or known drug effects:
  – Hepatic dysfunction may alter the way and the speed at which a drug is metabolized.
  – Renal dysfunction may alter drug excretion.
  – Vascular disease can affect the way a drug is absorbed and delivered to the tissues.
  – GI disorders can alter the way a drug is absorbed.
  – Pathologic conditions, such as heart failure, chronic lung disease, and endocrine disorders, can alter a drug's expected effects as well as the severity and seriousness of anticipated adverse effects.

Verifying the correct dose

When determining the correct dose of a particular drug for a particular patient, the prescriber must take into consideration the patient's weight, age, physical condition, and other drugs that the patient may be taking. However, it's important for the nurse to double-check these points before administering a drug, especially if the patient falls at the extreme in terms of age or weight, and to check the drug for specific warning signs or alerts. (See *Factors in verifying drug dosages*.)

PREVENT IT

*Medication error: On the chronic care unit, an elderly pa-
tient with a history of psychotic behavior was quite disorient-
ed and aggressive. It was decided to try quetiapine (Seroquel),
an antipsychotic, which had been used successfully in other
patients. He was started on the standard dosage—25 mg
orally twice daily—and this dose was increased to 50 mg
twice daily on the third day.*

*Within 2 days of the dose increase, the patient became de-
hydrated and tremulous and exhibited increased weakness
and sedation. The student nurse taking care of the patient
was required to prepare a care plan, including a detailed review of his drugs. She noted that elderly patients or patients
with hepatic impairment should be started on a lower than
normal dose of Seroquel and the dosage increased gradually.
She also noted from the patient's laboratory tests that he had
moderate hepatic dysfunction. When questioned, the prescriber reviewed the drug information and reduced the dose to
the starting level to see if the patient would improve.*

*Prevention: If a patient is at an extreme in age or weight,
always check the recommended dosage of a drug for additional guidelines. If a patient has liver or kidney dysfunction,
make a note on the patient's chart and check all drug dosages
against specific guidelines for these conditions. Being alert to
such potential problems can prevent serious errors.*

The nurse should also be alert for problems with
this particular drug, Seroquel.

IT'S A FACT

*There have been 17 reports of serious adverse reactions in-
volving mix-ups occurring between Serzone (nefazodone) and*

Seroquel. The errors were blamed on poor handwriting, look-alike bottles, and placement of these drugs next to each other on computer lists.

✦ Pediatric considerations

A child requires a different dose of most drugs than an adult. The "standard" dose listed in package inserts and in many reference books refers to the dose that's most effective for the adult male. Compared to an adult, a child may handle a drug differently with regard to all areas of pharmacokinetics — absorption, distribution, metabolism, and excretion. The responses of the child's organs to the effects of the drug may also vary because of the immaturity of the organs. Commonly, a child requires a smaller dose of a drug to achieve the comparable critical concentration. Rarely, a child may require a higher dose of a drug.

For ethical reasons, drug research isn't performed on children. Over time, however, enough information can be accumulated from experience with use of the drug to recommend a pediatric dosage. Drug guides include the pediatric dosage if this information is available. Sometimes a child may need a drug, but there's no recommended pediatric dosage for that particular drug. In such situations, there are established formulas for estimating the appropriate dosage. These methods of determining a pediatric dosage take into consideration the child's age, weight, or body surface area (BSA). (See *Conversion rules.*)

Perhaps the best approach to determining a child's dosage when no recommendation exists is to calculate the child's BSA, which incorporates height and weight. Using these measurements more closely reflects the child's growth and organ maturation. You can deter-

Conversion rules

Use one of the following conversion formulas to calculate the proper drug dosage for a pediatric patient:

✦ Fried's rule (for children under age 1) assumes that an adult dose would be appropriate for a child age 12½.

$$\text{dose (for a child} <1 \text{ year)} = \frac{\text{infant's age (in months)}}{150 \text{ months}} \times \text{average adult dose}$$

✦ Young's rule (for children age 1 to 12):

$$\text{dose (child 1 to 12 years)} = \frac{\text{child's age (in years)}}{\text{child's age (in years)} + 12} \times \text{average adult dose}$$

✦ Clark's rule assumes that the adult dose is based on a 150-lb (68-kg) person.

$$\text{child's dose} = \frac{\text{weight of child (lb)}}{150 \text{ lb}} \times \text{average adult dose}$$

mine a child's BSA by using a nomogram. (See *Reading a nomogram*, page 168.)

After the BSA is determined, this formula is then used to calculate the dose:

child's dose =
surface area in square meters × average adult dose 1.73.

With small children, even a tiny error can be critical. When working in pediatrics, it's important to become familiar with at least one of these conversion methods to determine a pediatric drug dose. Many facilities require that two nurses always check critical pediatric dosages. This is good practice when working with small children. Don't rely on the computer, the pharmacist, or the prescriber to calculate the correct dose.

Reading a nomogram

Body surface area (BSA) is critical when calculating drug doses for pediatric patients or doses that are extremely potent and must be given in precise amounts. The nomogram shown here lets you plot the patient's height and weight to determine the BSA. Here's how it works:

✦ Locate the patient's height in the left column of the nomogram and his weight in the right column.

✦ Use a ruler to draw a straight line connecting the two points. The point at which the line intersects the surface area column indicates the patient's BSA in square meters.

✦ For an average-size child, use the simplified nomogram in the box. Find the child's weight in pounds on the left side of the scale, and then read the corresponding BSA on the right side.

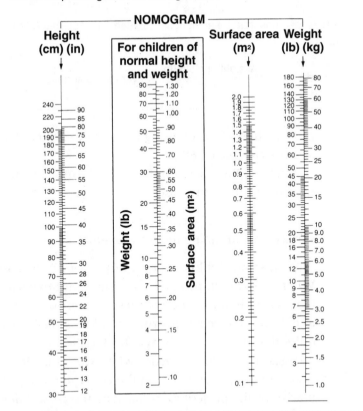

NOMOGRAM

Timesaving tips

When calculating safe pediatric doses, save time and prevent errors by following these suggestions:
✦ Carry a calculator to use when solving equations.
✦ Consult a formulary or drug guide to verify a drug dose. When in doubt, call the pharmacist.
✦ Keep the patient's weight in kilograms at his bedside so it is available quickly when needed.

The person administering the drug is responsible for assuring that the correct dose will be given. Always double-check the math before giving a drug this way. (See *Timesaving tips*.)

PREVENT IT

Medication error: A busy neurology fellow ordered phenobarbital (Barbita) 60 mg orally twice daily to prevent seizures in a 2-year-old child. The medication nurse for the day was unfamiliar with the use of phenobarbital in children and checked the drug before administering it. She found that the recommended range for phenobarbital in children was 3 to 6 mg/kg/day. She noted that the child weighed 22 lb (10 kg) on admission. Quickly checking the dosage range, she found that the recommended range was 30 to 60 mg per day — half of the prescribed order. She called the fellow who said that he had quickly used Clark's rule to determine the child's dose because he was more familiar with adult dosage ranges. Together, they rechecked the math as follows:

$$\text{child's dose} = 22 \text{ lb} \times (60 \text{ to } 100 \text{ mg/day})/150 \text{ lb} =$$
$$0.14 \times 60 \text{ to } 0.14 \times 100, \text{ or } 8 \text{ to } 14 \text{ mg/day}$$

This was remarkably different than the listed pediatric dosage. The fellow stated that he apparently had forgotten the actual formula to use and had calculated incorrectly. Researching further, they discovered that phenobarbital has a recommended pediatric dosage based on clinical experience and trials. Clark's rule shouldn't have been used in this situation. The order was rewritten for 60 mg per day in two divided doses.

Prevention: *When giving a drug to a child, always look it up in a reliable drug guide. If the guide doesn't list a recommended pediatric dosage, the best approach is to use a nomogram to determine the dose because this takes into account the child's weight and height and will more closely approximate growth and organ maturity. If a nomogram isn't available, use one of the conversion formulas, and always check the formula before doing the calculations. These formulas should be posted in pediatric areas for easy access. After doing the calculations, have another person check the math. Errors are common in math, especially when one is distracted or busy, so double-checking should be standard practice. A child is more susceptible to the effects and adverse effects of drugs and every precaution should be taken to ensure that the correct dose is used.*

✦ Availability considerations

Frequently, the dose that's needed for a child isn't what's available or provided. First, make sure that you check the medication's label for the actual dosage supplied. The label may be the right medication, but in a different dosage than was ordered. (See *Check that dosage!*)

Sometimes, only one dosage of the drug is available from the pharmacy or the drug is in a multiple-dose vial. Then the available dosage will need to be converted to the prescribed dose. Doing the mathematical cal-

Check that dosage!

The drug labels below show examples of a drug that you're likely to encounter in two different dosages. Carefully reading labels like these can help you avoid medication errors. The top label is Augmentin 200 mg/5 ml. The bottom label is Augmentin 400 mg/5 ml — twice the concentration of the other one.

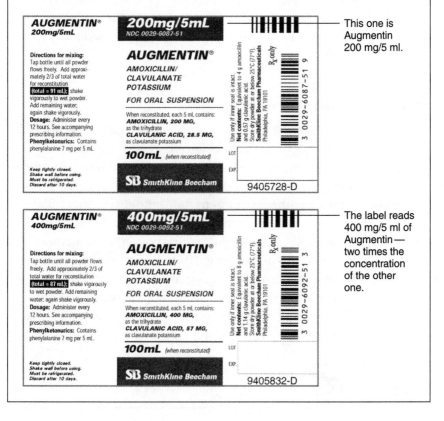

culations accurately is the shared responsibility of the prescriber who orders the drug, the pharmacist who dispenses it, and the nurse who administers it. This provides for multiple checks on the dose before the patient receives the drug.

In many facilities, drugs arrive at the patient care area in unit-dose form, prepackaged for an individual dose. Unwisely, the nurse administering the drug may rely on the prepackaged unit dose that's sent from the pharmacy and not even recalculate or recheck the dose against the written order. Mistakes happen, and the nurse, as the person administering the drug, is legally and professionally responsible for an error that occurs. Practicing nurses should know how to convert available forms of a drug into a specific drug dose to ensure that the patient receives the prescribed amount.

✦ Conversion considerations

To ensure that the patient receives what was ordered, it's a good idea to periodically review the various measurement systems. At least four different systems are used in drug preparation and delivery: metric system, apothecary system, household system, and avoirdupois system. With the growing number of drugs available and the increasing awareness of medication errors that occur daily, efforts have been made to decrease the number of systems in use in order to decrease the risk of errors that may occur as a result of converting between systems or misunderstanding abbreviations within systems.

IT'S A FACT

In 1995, the United States Pharmacopeia (USP) Convention established standards requiring that all prescriptions, regardless of the system used to calculate the drug dosage, include the metric measure for the drug quantity and strength. It also established that drugs would be dispensed only in the metric form.

Unfortunately, not all prescribers are totally in compliance with the USP standards, so nurses must be able to covert what's ordered into the available form to ensure patient safety. It's important to be able to perform conversions within each system of measure and between systems of measure. (See Measuring systems, *pages 174 and 175, and* Commonly used measures, *page 176.)*

The simplest way to convert measurements from one system to another is to set up a ratio and proportion equation, with the ratio containing two known equivalent amounts on one side of an equation and the ratio containing the amount you wish to convert and its unknown equivalent on the other side. To do this, first check a table of conversions to find out what the equivalent measure is in the two systems you're using. (See *Converting between systems,* page 177.)

Try the following conversion. Convert 6 fl oz (apothecary system) to the metric system of measure. According to the conversion table, 1 fl oz is equivalent to 30 ml. Use this information to set up a ratio:

$$\frac{1 \text{ fl oz}}{30 \text{ ml}} = \frac{6 \text{ fl oz}}{X}$$

The known ratio, 1 fl oz is equivalent to 30 ml, is on one side of the equation. The other side of the equation contains the amount you want to convert and its unknown equivalent, or X. Because fluid ounce is in the numerator (top number) on the left side of the equation, it must also be in the numerator on the right side of the equation. The above equation reads: 1 fl oz is to 30 ml as 6 fl oz are to how many milliliters?

The first step in this conversion is to cross-multiply:

$$\frac{1 \text{ fl oz}}{30 \text{ ml}} = \frac{6 \text{ fl oz}}{X}$$

Measuring systems

At least four different systems are currently used in drug preparation and delivery: metric, apothecary, household, and avoirdupois systems.

✦ *Metric system:* The most widely used system of measure, the metric system is based on the decimal system, so all units in the system are determined as multiples of 10. This system is used worldwide and makes it possible to share knowledge and research information. The metric system uses the gram as the basic unit of solid measure and the liter as the basic unit of liquid measure.

✦ *Apothecary system:* This old system of measure, specifically developed for use by apothecaries or pharmacists, uses the minim as the basic unit of liquid measure and the grain as the basic unit of solid measure. This system, more difficult to use than the metric system, is rarely used in clinical settings. Occasionally, however, a prescriber writes an order in this system, and the dosage has to be converted to an available form. This system has an interesting feature that causes confusion and errors: It uses roman numerals placed after the unit of measure to denote amounts. For example, 15 grains would be written "gr xv."

✦ *Household system:* This system, the one found in recipe books, uses the teaspoon as the basic unit of fluid measure and the grain as the basic unit of solid measure. Despite efforts in recent years to standardize measuring devices, wide variations have been noted in the capacity of some of these units. Patients should be advised that flatware teaspoons and drinking cups vary greatly in the volume they contain; for instance, a flatware teaspoon could hold up to 2 measuring teaspoons of quantity. When a patient is taking a liquid medication at home, it's important to clarify that the measures in the instructions refer to those obtained using standardized measuring devices.

✦ *Avoirdupois system:* Another older system that was very popular when pharmacists routinely had to compound medications themselves is the avoirdupois system. Seldom used by prescribers, the avoirdupois system may be used in bulk medication that comes directly from the manufacturer. If nurses need to become involved in preparing medications from bulk, special education programs should be available to explain this system and to test their ability to convert from this system appropriately.

Measuring systems *(continued)*

Some drugs are measured in other units. These measures may reflect chemical activity or biologic equivalence. One of these measures is the unit. A unit usually reflects the biologic activity of the drug in 1 ml of solution. The unit is unique to the drug it measures. A unit of heparin wouldn't be comparable to a unit of insulin.

Milliequivalents (mEq) are used to measure electrolytes (potassium, sodium, calcium, and fluoride). The mEq refers to the ionic activity of the drug. An order is usually written for a number of mEq, not a volume of drug.

International units are also sometimes used to measure certain vitamins or enzymes. These are also unique to each drug and can't be converted to other measuring forms.

If an order is written in a system that you aren't familiar with, ask the prescriber to specify exactly what's needed.

$$30 \text{ ml} \times 6 \text{ fl oz} = 1 \text{ fl oz} \times X$$

Using your algebra skills, you could also write this:

$$(30 \text{ ml})(6 \text{ fl oz}) = (1 \text{ fl oz}) X$$

Multiplying the numbers gives you:

$$180 \text{ (ml)(fl oz)} = 1 \text{ (fl oz)} X$$

Rearranging the terms to let the unknown stand alone on one side of the equation:

$$X = \frac{180 \text{ (ml)(fl oz)}}{1 \text{ (fl oz)}}$$

Whenever possible, cancel out numbers as well as units of measure. In the above equation, canceling out leaves:

$$X = 180 \text{ ml}$$

Commonly used measures

The following chart lists the most commonly used measures.

SYSTEM	SOLID MEASURE	LIQUID MEASURE
Metric	gram (g)	liter (L)
	1 milligram (mg) = 0.001 g	1 milliliter (ml) = 0.001 L
	1 microgram (µg) = 0.000001 g	1 ml = 1 cubic centimeter (cc)
	1 kilogram (kg) = 1,000 g	
Apothecary	grain (gr)	minim (min)
	60 gr = 1 dram (dr)	60 min = 1 fluidram (fl dr)
	8 dr = 1 ounce (oz)	8 fl dr = 1 fluid ounce (fl oz)
Household	pound (lb)	pint (pt)
	1 lb = 16 oz	2 pt = 1 quart (qt)
		4 qt = 1 gallon (gal)
		16 oz = 1 pt = 2 cups
		32 tablespoons (tbs) = 1 pt
		3 teaspoons (tsp) = 1 tbs

Canceling out the units of measure leaves you with the appropriate amount and unit of measure. The answer to the problem is that 6 fl oz is equivalent to 180 ml.

Converting between systems

The chart below presents accepted conversions between measurement systems. It's a good idea to post a conversion guide in the medication room or on the medication cart for easy access. When you use conversions frequently, remembering them is easy. However, when you don't use them frequently, the details may become fuzzy or lost—it's best to look them up.

METRIC	APOTHECARY	HOUSEHOLD
Solid measure		
1 kg		2.2 lb
454 kg		1.0 lb
1 g = 1,000 mg	15 gr (gr xv)	
60 mg	1 gr (gr i)	
30 mg	½ gr (gr ss)	
Liquid measure		
1 L = 1,000 ml		about 1 qt
240 ml	8 fl oz (fl oz viii)	1 C
30 ml	1 fl oz (fl oz i)	2 tbs
15 to 16 ml	4 fl dr (fl dr iv)	1 tbs = 3 tsp
8 ml	2 fl dr (fl dr ii)	2 tsp
4 to 5 ml	1 fl dr (fl dr i)	1 tsp = 60 gtt
1 ml	15 to 16 min (min xv or min xvi)	
0.06 ml	1 min (min i)	

Refresh your skills using another example. Convert 32 gr (apothecary) to the metric system, expressing the answer in mg. Find the conversion on the conversion table: 1 gr is equal to 60 mg. Set up the ratio.

$$\frac{1 \text{ gr}}{60 \text{ mg}} = \frac{32 \text{ gr}}{X}$$

$$1 \text{ gr } (X) = (32 \text{ gr})(60 \text{ mg})$$

$$1 \text{ gr } X = 1{,}920 \text{ (gr)(mg)}$$

$$X = \frac{1{,}920 \text{ (gr)(mg)}}{1 \text{ gr}}$$

$$X = 1{,}920 \text{ mg}$$

32 gr are equivalent to 1,920 mg.

PREVENT IT

Medication error: A visiting nurse needed to help a patient take 4 tablespoons (tbs) of Milk of Magnesia to prepare for an upcoming test. They looked through all of the household measures and found a teaspoon, but not a tablespoon. The nurse tried to recall how many teaspoons (tsp) were in 1 tbs and thought she remembered that there were two. She calculated that the patient would then need 8 tsp of Milk of Magnesia. When she got back to the office, she looked up the conversion and realized that the patient should have had 12 tsp because there are 3 tsp in 1 tbs.

Prevention: When left totally up to memory, conversions can cause errors. The nurse would have done well to call someone to check on the conversion, or even see if the patient had a cookbook that might list conversions within the household system. If you use a conversion all the time, it's easy to recall. If you haven't used a conversion for a while, look it up in a table. When in doubt, check it out. Luckily, the patient had no adverse effects from this error; with a different drug, it might have caused a problem.

✦ I.V. solution considerations

Verifying I.V. solutions is sometimes overlooked. They're commonly stocked with medication already added to them, usually potassium chloride (KCl). However, these solutions may be stocked with different strengths of KCl. Be sure to double-check the I.V. bag before hanging it to make sure it contains the right dose of additive. Also check the I.V. bag that is obtained from a stock bin — the bag may have been accidentally placed in the wrong bin.

When assuming care of a patient, always check that the I.V. solution that is infusing is the one that was ordered. Sometimes I.V. orders are changed and the nurse isn't aware of it, consequently, the I.V. solution isn't changed and, technically, the patient is receiving the wrong dose of medication.

Total parenteral nutrition (TPN) also presents a concern. This nutritional I.V. infusion commonly includes many additives that are ordered specifically for the patient according to laboratory values. Be sure to check all the ingredients against the order before hanging the bag. Don't assume that the pharmacy mixed it correctly. Some facilities have a specific procedure for hanging TPN bags to avoid errors.

PREVENT IT

Medication error: *Judy Robinson, a 50-year-old trauma victim, was receiving TPN. On the weekend evening shift, a* *per diem nurse was caring for her. It was the usual busy unit, with visitors and dinner coinciding. It was time for Mrs. Robinson's TPN to be changed—in fact, the infusion bag had run dry. The nurse grabbed the premixed TPN bag from the refrigerator and quickly started it.*

Two hours later, Mrs. Robinson was diaphoretic, tachycardiac, and restless. Further assessment revealed that her blood sugar was dangerously low at 49. Measures were taken to correct the blood sugar. It was discovered that the TPN infusion contained 100 units of insulin instead of the 10 units ordered for this patient. The TPN was discontinued and an I.V. solution of 10% dextrose and water was infused until the correct TPN solution could be prepared.

Prevention: *This error could have been prevented if the nurse had compared the physician's order against the ingredients in the TPN bag. The nurse assumed that the TPN solution was correct because it had the correct name on the bag. TPN contains several ingredients, ordered specifically for a patient's needs. All the ingredients should be checked every time an infusion bag is changed.*

✦ Calculating the correct dose

As previously mentioned, there are several measurement systems available that may be used when a drug is ordered. Because drugs are made available only in certain forms or doses, it may become necessary to calculate what a patient should receive when you interpret a drug order. Generally, if the units to be administered are equivalent to more than 1 or 2 available units, the dose should be recalculated. A patient shouldn't have to take 5 or 10 tablets to receive a therapeutic dose. Whenever you have to give a lot of oral medication or use multiple vials, an alarm should go off. If you calculate a dose and need a large number of available units, recalculate that dose. If you still come up with a large number of units, check the original order. You may be working with the wrong drug or a misread dose. Then go one step further and have another nurse or pharmacist check your calculation before administering the drug

Calculating tablets or capsules

Tablets or capsules for oral administration may not be available in the prescribed dose. In these situations, the nurse administering the drug must calculate the number of tablets or capsules that must be given to achieve the ordered dose.

The easiest way to determine this is to set up a ratio of proportion equation. The ratio containing the two known equivalent amounts is put on one side of the equation and the ratio containing the unknown value is put on the other side. The known equivalent is the amount of drug available in one tablet or capsule; the unknown is the number of tablets or capsules that will be needed to administer the prescribed dose:

$$\frac{\text{amount of drug available}}{\text{one tablet/capsule}} = \frac{\text{amount of drug prescribed}}{\text{number of tablets/}\atop\text{capsules to give}}$$

Try this example: An order is written for 10 gr of aspirin (which is written as *gr X, aspirin*). The available tablets each contain 5 gr. How many tablets should be administered to achieve the prescribed dose?

$$\frac{5 \text{ gr}}{1 \text{ tablet}} = \frac{10 \text{ gr}}{X}$$

Cross-multiply the ratio:

$$5 \text{ (gr)}X = 10 \text{ (gr)(tablet)}$$

Solve for X. Rearrange and cancel units and numbers:

$$X = \frac{10\ (gr)(tablet)}{5\ (gr)}$$

$$X = 2\ tablets$$

Try another example: An order is written for 0.05 g oral spironolactone (Aldactone). The spironolactone is available in 25-mg tablets. How many tablets are needed?

First, convert the grams to milligrams. To do this, check the conversion table which shows that 1 g is equivalent to 1,000 mg, and set up a proportion ratio:

$$\frac{1\ g}{1,000\ mg} = \frac{0.05\ g}{X}$$

Cross-multiply:

$$1\ (g)\ X = 0.05\ (g) \times 1000\ (mg)$$

Simplify:

$$X = \frac{50\ (g)(mg)}{1\ (g)}$$

$$X = 50\ mg$$

Now the order is converted to the same measurement as the available tablets. Next, solve for the number of tablets that are required to achieve the prescribed dose:

$$\frac{25\ mg}{1\ tablet} = \frac{50\ mg}{desired\ dose}$$

$$desired\ dose\ (25\ mg) = 50\ (mg)(tablet)$$

$$desired\ dose = \frac{50\ (mg)(tablet)}{25\ mg}$$

$$\text{desired dose} = 2 \text{ tablets}$$

This is relatively simple math; it just takes practice. Relying on unit-dose or other systems to determine the correct unit delivery calls for less mathematical skill, and calculation practice may be less necessary. However, it's advisable to always to double-check the dose and units before administering a drug.

PREVENT IT

Medication error: *An order was written for a patient to take 0.75 g of oral tetracycline (Panmycin) to be started immediately. The nurse found that the drug was available only in 250-mg tablets in the floor stock. She quickly did a mental calculation and determined that the patient should be getting 30 tablets per day. Assuming that the drug would be available in larger concentrations from the pharmacy, she didn't check her math but gave the patient 15 tablets to start, making a note for the evening nurse to give the other half of the order with the evening medications.*

The evening nurse had never seen a request for 15 tablets and decided to check the order. Referring to a drug guide, she found that the prescribed dose was standard. She checked the bottle in the floor stock and found that it was 250 mg; she then recalculated the number of tablets needed and came up with 3, not 30. She had another nurse check her calculations:

$$\frac{250 \text{ mg}}{\text{tablet}} = \frac{0.75}{X}$$

She checked the conversion table and found that 0.75 g was equivalent to 750 mg.

$$\frac{250 \text{ mg}}{\text{tablet}} = \frac{750 \text{ mg}}{X}$$

$$250 \text{ (mg) X} = 750 \text{ (mg) tablets}$$

$$X = 3 \text{ tablets}$$

Prevention: *The next day, the nurse-manager reviewed the error with the nurse who calculated the original dose. She had determined that 0.75 g was equal to 75 mg and that's how she had gotten off track. They reviewed the conversion table that was posted, and it was decided that a second nurse should always recheck math when a dose needed to be calculated. Generally, if a patient needed 30 tablets to receive the prescribed dose, it should have set off alerts that there was an error somewhere—wrong drug, wrong dosage, or wrong calculation.*

Sometimes, the desired dose will be a fraction of a tablet or capsule, one-half or one-quarter. Some tablets come with score markings that allow them to be cut. Pill cutters are readily available in most pharmacies to help patients cut tablets appropriately at home. However, one must use caution when advising a patient to cut a tablet. Many tablets today come in a matrix system that allows for slow and steady release of the active drug. These drugs can't be cut, crushed, or chewed. If the only way to deliver the correct dose to the patient is by cutting these preparations, a different drug or approach to treating the patient should be used.

PREVENT IT

Medication error: *Mr. Jones was diagnosed with cellulitis caused by Staphylococcus aureus. He was given a prescription for cefaclor (Ceclor) 250 mg orally every 8 hours. On the way home, his wife reminded him that she had been taking the* *same drug for acute bronchitis and was sure they had some left over. When they checked, her prescription was for Ceclor CD, 500 mg. With a pill cutter, they cut her tablets in half to save the money of filling another prescription.*

Later that night, Mr. Jones became dizzy and nauseous. He later developed abdominal pain and diarrhea. The couple became concerned that the pills may have "gone bad" and called the physician to explain what had happened. The physician asked them to come in immediately and to bring the bottle and the new prescription script with them. The pill that was cut in half was in an extended-release matrix; cutting the pill destroyed the delivery system, giving the patient the full dose of the drug all at once. The physician asked them to throw away the leftover pills, and then educated them about the importance of completing the full prescription and not saving drugs. He explained that the emergence of many drug-resistant strains stemmed from the failure to complete full drug prescriptions.

Prevention: *Several errors combined to cause this problem. The patient figured out the dose he needed to fill his prescription based on an "apples and oranges" effect. A drug in an extended-release form isn't the same as one that isn't. Every time the patient and his wife were given a prescription for an antibiotic, they should have been instructed on the importance of completing the course of the drug, even after they started to feel better. Unfortunately, with the high cost of prescription medications, many people tend to do this to save money or to self-treat if they get sick again. In this case, the math was right, but the dosage was inappropriate for the drug used.*

Calculating liquid preparations

Many drugs come in liquid form for a child or for an adult who may have difficulty swallowing a pill or tablet. Some drugs that don't come in a liquid can be prepared as a liquid by the pharmacist. If a patient is unable to swallow a tablet or capsule, check for other available forms and consult with the pharmacist about the possibility of preparing the drug in a liquid form. The same principle used to determine the number of tablets needed to achieve the prescribed dose can be used to determine the volume of the liquid needed to administer the prescribed dose. The ratio on the left of the equation is the known equivalents, and the right side of the ratio contains the unknown. The phrase "amount of drug" must appear in the numerator of both ratios.

$$\frac{\text{amount of drug available}}{\text{volume available}} = \frac{\text{amount of drug prescribed}}{\text{volume to administer}}$$

Try this example: An order has been written for 250 mg sulfisoxazole (Gantrisin). The bottle states that the solution contains 125 mg/5 ml. How much of the liquid should be given to achieve the prescribed dose?

$$\frac{125 \text{ mg}}{5 \text{ ml}} = \frac{250 \text{ mg}}{\text{desired dose}}$$

Cross-multiply:

$$125 \text{ (mg) desired dose} = 250 \text{ (mg)} \times 5 \text{ (ml)}$$

Simplify:

$$\text{desired dose} = \frac{1250 \text{ (mg)(ml)}}{125 \text{ mg}}$$

$$\text{desired dose} = 10 \text{ ml}$$

Even if the facility provides unit-dose medications, calculate the dose to give. This is a skill that everyone who administers drugs should have.

PREVENT IT

Medication error: A busy medication nurse on a surgical unit was asked to medicate a patient who had undergone a radical neck resection and was in severe pain. Checking the medication record, the nurse saw an order for 20 mg of liquid morphine sulfate via nasogastric tube every 3 hours as needed, and the last dose had been given more than 3 hours ago. She took the bottle labeled "morphine sulfate 20 mg/5 ml," poured out the dose in the calibrated plastic cup, and immediately administered it to the patient. Because the patient was in such distress, the nurse didn't double-check the dose and assumed that she had compared the bottle and dose.

Shortly after the patient had received the drug, his primary nurse reported that his respiratory rate was decreasing and he was difficult to arouse. After checking for bleeding or other problems, the nurse questioned the pain medication order. The medication nurse checked the orders, compared them with the medication record, and checked the label of the bottle. She then realized that she had given the patient 20 ml of the drug instead of 20 mg. She had confused mg and ml and had actually given the patient 80 mg of morphine, not 20 mg:

$$\frac{\text{amount of drug available}}{\text{volume available}} = \frac{\text{amount of drug prescribed}}{\text{volume to administer}}$$

$$\frac{20 \text{ mg}}{5 \text{ ml}} = \frac{20 \text{ mg}}{X}$$

$$20 \text{ mg}(X) = 100 \text{ mg(ml)}$$

$$X = 5 \text{ ml}$$

The nurse hadn't carefully checked the math before giving the drug to the patient and quickly poured 20 ml into the cup instead of the 5 ml she should have used. The attending physician was quickly notified, and naloxone (Narcan) was ad-

*ministered to counteract the effects of the morphine. The pa-
tient was closely monitored and recovered without incident.*

*   **Prevention:** *Every time that preparing a medication requires calculation, make sure that you double-check the order,
the available form, and your math. If you are rushed or
stressed or it seems like a routine calculation that you can do
in your head, step back and take a second to review what
you're doing. If the nurse had taken a few seconds to carefully
calculate the dose in this case or had had another nurse check
her calculations, she would have saved several hours of intense nursing care, paperwork, and potential patient problems. Prevention is the best medicine. Always calculate the
dose and always double-check.*

A problem reported repeatedly in home care situations involves errors in measuring liquid drugs to
achieve the right dose. When an order is written for
1 tsp of a liquid drug, it's referring to the teaspoon designated in the household system of measure, which is
5 ml of solution.

IT'S A FACT

*The capacity of teaspoons found in typical tableware sets can
range from 3.75 to 7.5 ml. Many pharmacies sell measuring
devices or may supply them when they fill prescriptions for
liquid medications. Without proper instruction, however, the
patient may still use the everyday tableware as a measuring
device.*

If a patient is told to take 1 tsp of a drug, it's critical
to teach the patient that it means one measuring teaspoon, not a teaspoon from his tableware set. If a patient uses a tableware teaspoon to measure the dose,

he could overdose or underdose and not receive the desired therapeutic effect.

PREVENT IT

Medication error: Five-year-old Jenna was seen in the ED for an acute asthma attack. At discharge, she was given a prescription for albuterol (Ventolin), 2 mg/5 ml, 150 ml: sig: 1 tsp P.O. t.i.d. Her father had the prescription filled at the pharmacy and was told that Jenna should be given 1 tsp three times per day. Four days later, Jenna was brought into the ED again. She was in moderate distress, pale, diaphoretic, and restless with a pulse rate of 148 beats/minute, blood pressure of 118/60 mm Hg, respirations of 28 breaths/minute, and an oxygen saturation of 93%. It was clear that she wasn't having another asthma attack. Her presentation was consistent with albuterol toxicity.

Jenna was hydrated with normal saline and monitored. Her distraught parents had her medication with them and the nurse was surprised to see that the bottle was well over one-half gone in 4 days. The parents told the nurse that they shook the bottle well before each use and poured out a teaspoon for Jenna to take. They couldn't understand how she could have received too much medication. The nurse inquired what kind of teaspoon was used, and they explained that they just used an ordinary teaspoon. When they returned the next day to take Jenna home, they brought in the teaspoon they were using and found that it had a capacity of 7.5 ml. Jenna was receiving 50% more than the prescribed dose each time she took the drug. Jenna's parents were shocked and said that no one had told them that they should use a specific device or that a measuring teaspoon might be different from a table-ware teaspoon.

Prevention: Use of oral liquid medications is increasing. Although young children commonly receive a liquid drug, more older children and elderly adults are also receiving liq-

Looking at combination drugs

Before taking on complex dose computations, take a quick look at this drug label. As it states, Septra contains 40 mg of trimethoprim and 200 mg of sulfamethoxazole. Instead of ordering it with a two-part dosage, the physician prescribes the trade name Septra and the volume of elixir to be given.

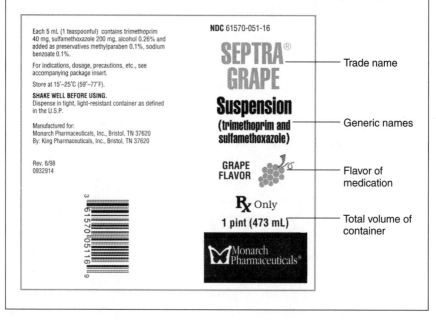

Each 5 mL (1 teaspoonful) contains trimethoprim 40 mg, sulfamethoxazole 200 mg, alcohol 0.26% and added as preservatives methylparaben 0.1%, sodium benzoate 0.1%.

For indications, dosage, precautions, etc., see accompanying package insert.

Store at 15°–25°C (59°–77°F).

SHAKE WELL BEFORE USING.
Dispense in tight, light-resistant container as defined in the U.S.P.

Manufactured for:
Monarch Pharmaceuticals, Inc., Bristol, TN 37620
By: King Pharmaceuticals, Inc., Bristol, TN 37620

Rev. 6/98
0932914

NDC 61570-051-16

SEPTRA® GRAPE — Trade name

Suspension
(trimethoprim and sulfamethoxazole) — Generic names

GRAPE FLAVOR — Flavor of medication

R Only

1 pint (473 mL) — Total volume of container

Monarch Pharmaceuticals®

uid because of difficulty swallowing pills. Health care providers are usually very careful with parent education in giving small children a liquid drug, usually providing special syringes or measuring devices to assure that patients receive the right dose. Older children and adults commonly don't receive special instructions or measuring devices.

Education is the key to preventing this medication error. One ED used this typical error as a basis for a staff education program. Each staff member brought in a teaspoon from home, and they were amazed to see the variation in capacities of these teaspoons. This educational program left a lasting im-

pression on the physicians and nurses, who were then very careful to explain using a measuring teaspoon to their patients. Notices were posted on bulletin boards in the patient waiting area and staff room to remind patients and staff about how to ensure the right dose of a liquid medication.

Calculating combination drugs

Certain medications may contain two drugs. The labels for these combination drugs contain the generic names of both drugs and their doses. These drugs are ordered by their trade names and the amount of the drugs to be given. (See *Looking at combination drugs.*)

Calculating parenteral drugs

Before you give a parenteral (by injection) drug, be sure to read the label closely. Some of these medications are dispensed in multiple-dose vials. Careful examination of the label helps the nurse calculate, prepare, and administer the correct dose. (See *Looking at labels,* page 192.)

Drugs administered parenterally must be given in liquid form. If the drug needs to be prepared, examine the label for information on correctly mixing the drug to obtain the right dose. However, you may need the package insert for such instructions. (See *Looking at inserts,* page 193.)

After the drug is prepared correctly, the person administering it needs to calculate the volume necessary for the correct dose. The same formula can be used for this calculation as is used to determine the dose of an oral liquid drug.

$$\frac{\text{amount of drug available}}{\text{volume available}} = \frac{\text{amount of drug prescribed}}{\text{volume to administer}}$$

Looking at labels

The labels below show all the information you need to safely administer a parenteral drug. Read them carefully!

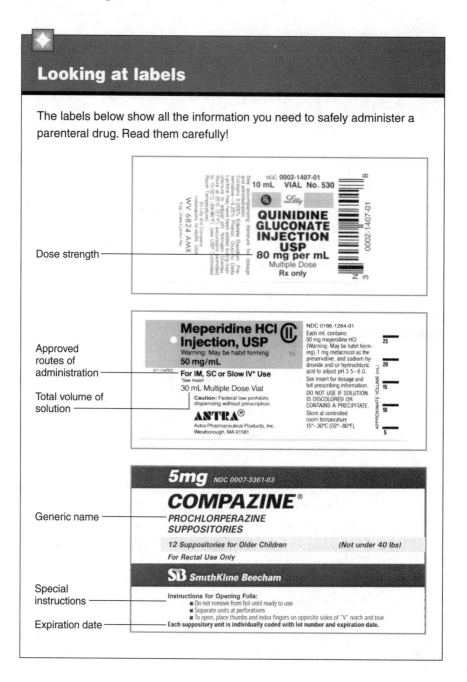

Dose strength

Approved routes of administration

Total volume of solution

Generic name

Special instructions

Expiration date

Looking at inserts

Package inserts included with drugs commonly provide information that may not be on the outer labels. For example, although the drug label for ceftazidime provides no information about reconstitution, the package insert does. Here are the possible diluent combinations as they appear in the package insert that comes with this drug:

VIAL SIZE	DILUENT TO BE ADDED	APPROXIMATE AVAILABLE	APPROXIMATE AVERAGE CONCENTRATION
I.M. or I.V. direct (bolus) injection			
1 g	3 ml	3.6 ml	280 mg/ml
I.V. infusion			
1 g	10 ml	10.6 ml	95 mg/ml
2 g	10 ml	11.2 ml	180 mg/ml

Try this example: An order was written for 75 mg meperidine (Demerol) intramuscularly. The vial states that it contains meperidine 50 mg per 1 ml.

Set up the equation as you did earlier:

$$\frac{50 \text{ mg}}{1 \text{ ml}} = \frac{75 \text{ mg}}{\text{desired dose}}$$

$$50 \text{ (mg) desired dose} = 75 \text{ (mg) (ml)}$$

$$\text{desired dose} = \frac{75 \text{ (mg)(ml)}}{50 \text{ mg}}$$

$$\text{desired dose} = 1.5 \text{ ml}$$

1.5 ml of the meperidine is the correct amount to administer to achieve the prescribed dose.

PREVENT IT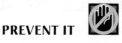

Medication error: *A patient came into the ED in acute distress related to an asthma episode. The attending physician prescribed aminophylline (Phyllocontin) 100 mg I.V. to be started as soon as possible. The nurse went to the floor stock and found the vial for aminophylline, 500 mg/2.5 ml. She mentally calculated that the patient should receive a 5-ml injection. She prepared the injection and gave it to the physician to administer. Puzzled at the 5-ml injection, the physician asked the nurse to recheck the dosage. Flustered, the nurse went back to the floor stock, got the bottle, and asked a colleague to calculate the required dosage with her:*

$$\frac{\text{amount of drug available}}{\text{volume available}} = \frac{\text{amount of drug prescribed}}{\text{volume to administer}}$$

$$\frac{500 \text{ mg}}{2.5 \text{ ml}} = \frac{100 \text{ mg}}{\text{desired dose (X)}}$$

$$500 \text{ mg (X)} = 250 \text{ mg (ml)}$$

$$X = 0.5 \text{ ml}$$

Both nurses rechecked the math several times. Both agreed that the actual dose should have been 0.5 ml, and not 5 ml. A new syringe was prepared, and the patient received the correct amount. The physician stated that he also had problems with dose calculations, but because he had given this drug so often, the large amount in the syringe appeared to be incorrect.

Prevention: *Always write out a dosage calculation to be sure it's correct. This can save time in the long run and prevent potentially serious medication errors.*

Calculating decimal point conversions

Many calculation errors involve decimal points. It's easy to place the decimal point in the wrong place, which could mean a dose that's 10, 100, or 1,000 times greater or less than the prescribed dosage.

PREVENT IT

Medication error: Heparin, 800 units, is ordered for a patient. The heparin is supplied in a multiple-dose vial that's labeled 10,000 units/ml. A student nurse taking care of a patient was asked to draw up the heparin and administer it. The student wrote out the formula and calculated the dose as follows:

$$\frac{\text{amount of drug available}}{\text{volume available}} = \frac{\text{amount of drug prescribed}}{\text{volume to administer}}$$

$$\frac{10,000 \text{ units}}{\text{ml}} = \frac{800 \text{ units}}{\text{desired dose (X)}}$$

$$10,000 \text{ units (X)} = 800 \text{ units/ml}$$

$$X = 0.8 \text{ ml}$$

The student nurse drew up the heparin and took it to her instructor for verification, along with the calculation. After a review, the instructor asked her to redo the math. She still came up with 0.8 ml. Then, the instructor gave her a "quick check" tip for verifying calculations: Multiply the answer you came up with by the available units and see if you then come up with the ordered dose:

$$0.8 \text{ ml} \times 10,000 \text{ units} = 8,000 \text{ units}$$

The student had calculated a dose that was 10 times the prescribed amount. She was upset because the more she double-checked her math, the more convinced she became that she was correct.

> *Prevention:* Whenever a math calculation involves determining a drug dose — especially if decimal points are involved — double-check the math. It's safer if someone else can check it as well because when an error occurs, it's typically difficult to detect it yourself. The instructor's "quick check" tip is a good safety net if you can't get a second opinion on your calculations. Multiply the amount you have decided to give with the available concentration, and you should get the prescribed dose.

Calculating I.V. solutions

I.V. solutions are used to deliver a prescribed amount of fluid, electrolytes, vitamins, nutrients, or drugs directly into the bloodstream. Although there's less room for error when administering I.V. drugs, it's important to be certain that the dose you're administering is what was prescribed. Most facilities now use electronically monitored delivery systems; however, it's still important to use standard calculations to determine the amount of an I.V. solution that needs to be given.

Most I.V. delivery systems have a standard control called a microdrip in which each milliliter delivered contains 60 drops. Although macrodrop systems — which deliver 15 drops/ml — are also available, they're usually used when a large volume needs to be delivered quickly. The microdrop system is most commonly used when drugs are given I.V. Check the packaging of the I.V. tubing if you have doubts or are unfamiliar with the equipment.

The ratio that's used to determine how many drops of fluid you'll be administering per minute is:

$$\text{drops/minute} = \frac{\text{ml of solution prescribed/hour} \times \text{drops delivered/ml}}{60 \text{ minutes/hour}}$$

The drops per minute—or the rate you'll set by adjusting the valve on the I.V. tubing—is equal to the amount of solution that has been prescribed per hour multiplied by the number of drops delivered per milliliter, then divided by 60 minutes in 1 hour.

Try this example: An order has been written for a patient to receive 400 ml of dextrose 5% in water (D_5W) over 4 hours. Calculate the drops per minute setting.

$$\text{drops/minute} = \frac{400 \text{ ml/4 hours} \times 60 \text{ drops/ml}}{60 \text{ minutes/hour}}$$

Simplify:

$$\text{drops/minute} = \frac{100 \text{ ml/hour} \times 60 \text{ drops/ml}}{60 \text{ minutes/hour}}$$

$$\text{drops/minute} = \frac{6{,}000 \text{ drops/hour}}{60 \text{ minutes/hour}}$$

$$\text{drops/minute} = 100$$

Calculating the same order for an I.V. set that delivers 15 drops/minute:

$$\text{drops/minute} = \frac{400 \text{ ml/4 hours} \times 15 \text{ drops/ml}}{60 \text{ minutes/hour}}$$

Simplify:

$$\text{drops/minute} = \frac{100 \text{ ml/hour} \times 15 \text{ drops/ml}}{60 \text{ minutes/hour}}$$

$$\text{drops/minute} = \frac{1{,}500 \text{ drops/hour}}{60 \text{ minutes/hour}}$$

$$\text{drops/minute} = 25$$

If a patient has an order for a drug to be given in an I.V. solution, the drug may first need to be mixed in a

Looking at piggyback infusions

An I.V. piggyback is a small-volume, intermittent infusion that's connected to an existing I.V. line containing maintenance fluid. Most piggybacks contain antibiotics or electrolytes. To calculate piggyback infusions, use proportions.

PIGGYBACK PROBLEM

You receive an order for 500 mg of imipenem in 100 ml of normal saline solution to be infused over 1 hour. The imipenem vial contains 1,000 mg (1 g). The insert says to reconstitute the powder with 5 ml of normal saline solution. How much solution should you draw? What is the flow rate?

SOLUTION SOLUTION

Write the first ratio to describe the known solution strength (amount of drug compared with the known amount of solution):

1,000 mg : 5 ml

✦ Write the second ratio, which compares the desired dose of imipenem and the unknown amount of solution:

500 mg : X

✦ Put these ratios into a proportion:
1,000 mg : 5 ml : : 500 mg : X

✦ Multiply the extremes and the means:
1,000 mg $\times$ X = 500 mg $\times$ 5 ml

✦ Solve for X by dividing each side of the equation by 1,000 mg and canceling units that appear in the numerator and denominator:

$$\frac{1,000 \text{ mg} \times X}{1,000 \text{ mg}} = \frac{500 \text{ mg} \times 5 \text{ ml}}{1,000 \text{ mg}}$$

$$X = \frac{500 \times 5 \text{ ml}}{1,000}$$

$$X = \frac{2,500 \text{ ml}}{1,000}$$

$$X = 2.5 \text{ ml}$$

You should draw up 2.5 ml of solution to get 500 mg of imipenem.

FLOW RATE

Recall that the flow rate is the number of milliliters of fluid to administer over 1 hour.

Looking at piggyback infusions *(continued)*

COMPATIBILITY COUNTS

After you've calculated an I.V. piggyback dose, make sure that the drugs to be infused together are compatible. This applies to drugs mixed in the same syringe or I.V. bag. Drug compatibility charts can be time-savers; you should have one hanging in your unit's medication room. If not, use a drug guide that includes a compatibility chart.

solution, which necessitates the first calculation. After the solution is mixed, apply the same principle as explained above to calculate the speed of the delivery. (See *Looking at piggyback infusions.*)

For example: An order is written for a patient to receive 50 ml of an antibiotic over 30 minutes. The I.V. set used is the 60 drop/ml, which allows greater control.

Calculate the appropriate speed of the delivery system.

$$\text{drops/minute} = \frac{50 \text{ ml/0.5 hours} \times 60 \text{ drops/ml}}{60 \text{ minutes/hour}}$$

Simplify:

$$\text{drops/minute} = \frac{100 \text{ ml/hour} \times 60 \text{ drops/ml}}{60 \text{ minutes/hour}}$$

$$\text{drops/minute} = \frac{6{,}000 \text{ drops/hour}}{60 \text{ minutes/hour}}$$

$$\text{drops/minute} = 100$$

PREVENT IT

Medication error: A nurse on orientation needed to start an
I.V. solution of 1,000 ml of normal saline to infuse over 10
hours. She checked the drop factor on the package of I.V. tubing and it stated 15 drops/ml. Using the formula that had
just been reviewed in the orientation program, the nurse calculated:

$$\text{drops/minute} = \frac{\text{ml of solution prescribed/hour} \times \text{drops delivered/ml}}{60 \text{ minutes/hour}}$$

$$\text{drops/minute} = \frac{1{,}000 \text{ ml/hour} \times 15 \text{ drops/ml}}{60 \text{ minutes/hour}}$$

$$\text{drops/minute} = \frac{15{,}000 \text{ drops/hour}}{60 \text{ minutes/hour}}$$

$$\text{drops/minute} = 250$$

*The nurse wasn't able to count 250 drops/minute and asked
the floor nurse, who was acting as her mentor, for assistance.
The floor nurse reviewed her calculations and they appeared
accurate. Although she got the same answer when she
worked the problem, she knew from experience that they always ran this order at 25 drops/minute. Frustrated, they
asked the nurse-manager, who had been teaching the orientation class, to review the problem with them. She looked at
the problem the way that they had set it up, compared it with
the order, and immediately saw that they had used the formula correctly but neglected to include that the order was
written for 10 hours, not 1 hour. Using that information, they
recalculated:*

$$\text{drops/minute} = \frac{\text{ml of solution prescribed/hour} \times \text{drops delivered/ml}}{60 \text{ minutes/hour}}$$

$$\text{drops/minute} = \frac{1{,}000 \text{ ml}/10 \text{ hours} \times 15 \text{ drops/ml}}{60 \text{ minutes/hour}}$$

$$\text{drops/minute} = \frac{1{,}500 \text{ drops/hour}}{60 \text{ minutes/hour}}$$

$$\text{drops/minute} = 25$$

The I.V. tubing was adjusted to deliver 25 drops/minute.

Prevention: *The patient didn't have a problem in this situation because the nurse had doubts when she calculated the amount of drug to deliver. When in doubt, check it out. When she double-checked her own calculations and couldn't get a different answer, she asked a colleague to check. When they both had doubts, they kept checking. Although it's easy to make a math error, it can be very difficult to find it when you keep repeating the problem. The math was correct in this case; however, the formula was not used correctly because the 10 hours was not considered in the original calculation. Always remember to double-check the math. If a conversion chart is available, it may be a good idea also to double-check your results against the chart. (See* Drip rate guide, *pages 202 and 203.)*

Calculating continuous medication infusions

Some drugs need to be diluted in I.V. solutions and administered carefully at a specific rate to achieve the desired effect. Many drugs come from the pharmacy premixed and ready to administer. In other situations, especially in emergency situations in the ICU or ED, the nurse needs to quickly determine how much drug to dilute in the I.V. solution and how fast to deliver the drug to the patient. The same process should be used to make these determinations.

Drip rate guide

When calculating the drip rate of I.V. solutions, remember that the number of drops required to deliver 1 ml varies with the type of administration set and the manufacturer. To calculate the drip rate, you need to know the drip factor for each product. As a quick reference, consult the chart below.

MANUFACTURER	DRIP FACTOR	DROPS/MINUTE TO INFUSE (DRIP RATE)	
		500 ml/24 hours	1,000 ml/24 hours
		21 ml/hour	42 ml/hour
Abbott	15 gtt/ml	5 gtt	10 gtt
Baxter-Healthcare	10 gtt/ml	3 gtt	7 gtt
Cutter	20 gtt/ml	7 gtt	14 gtt
IVAC	20 gtt/ml	7 gtt	14 gtt
McGaw	15 gtt/ml	5 gtt	10 gtt

First, you'll need to determine the concentration of the drug in the solution you're using:

$$\text{concentration in mg/ml} = \frac{\text{mg of the drug being used}}{\text{ml of I.V. solution}}$$

Then you'll need to figure out the flow rate you'll need to deliver the desired dose of the drug:

$$\frac{\text{dose in mg/minute}}{\text{dose to deliver/minute}} = \frac{\text{concentration in mg/ml}}{1 \text{ ml of solution}}$$

Try this example: A patient was admitted to the ED with chest pain and was having runs of a ventricular arrhythmia. An order was written to add 2 g or

1,000 ml/20 hours	1,000 ml/10 hours	1,000 ml/8 hours	1,000 ml/6 hours
50 ml/hour	100 ml/hour	125 ml/hour	166 ml/hour
12 gtt	25 gtt	31 gtt	42 gtt
8 gtt	17 gtt	21 gtt	28 gtt
17 gtt	34 gtt	42 gtt	56 gtt
17 gtt	34 gtt	42 gtt	56 gtt
12 gtt	25 gtt	31 gtt	42 gtt

2,000 mg of lidocaine to 500 ml of D_5W to infuse at 2 mg/minute.

First, figure out the concentration of the prepared solution:

$$\text{concentration in mg/ml} = \frac{\text{mg of the drug being used}}{\text{ml of I.V. solution}}$$

$$\text{concentration} = \frac{2,000 \text{ mg}}{500 \text{ ml}}$$

$$\text{concentration} = 4 \text{ mg/ml}$$

Then, figure out the flow rate to use to deliver the desired dose:

$$\frac{\text{dose in mg/minute}}{\text{dose to deliver/minute}} = \frac{\text{concentration in mg/ml}}{1 \text{ ml of solution}}$$

$$\frac{2 \text{ mg/ml}}{X} = \frac{4 \text{ mg/ml}}{1 \text{ ml}}$$

$$X \ (4 \text{ mg/ml}) = 2 \text{ mg}$$

$$X = \frac{2 \text{ mg}}{4 \text{ mg/ml}}$$

$$X = 0.5 \text{ ml}$$

To deliver the ordered dose of 2 mg/minute, you need to give the patient 0.5 ml/minute. If you're counting drops using a microdrip system, you would use the calculations you used earlier to determine the I.V. rate:

$$\text{drops/minute} = \frac{\text{ml of solution prescribed/hour} \times \text{drops delivered/ml}}{60 \text{ minutes/hour}}$$

The drops per minute, or the rate you'll set by adjusting the valve on the I.V. tubing, is equal to the amount of solution that has been prescribed per hour multiplied by the number of drops delivered per milliliter divided by 60 minutes in 1 hour.

First, convert the dose per minute to dose per hour by multiplying by 60 because there are 60 minutes in 1 hour:

$$0.5 \text{ ml/minute} \times 60 \text{ minutes} = 30 \text{ ml}$$

Now calculate the drops per minute setting:

$$\text{drops/minute} = \frac{30 \text{ ml/hour} \times 60 \text{ drops/ml}}{60 \text{ minutes/hour}}$$

Simplify:

$$\text{drops/minute} = \frac{1,800 \text{ drops/hour}}{60 \text{ minutes/hour}}$$

$$\text{drops/minute} = 30$$

If you're using an I.V. infusion system, you'll set the system to deliver 30 drops per minute.

Sometimes, the dosing of these drugs is so critical that the orders are written based on the patient's weight. The order may be written for a dose of drug per each kilogram of weight per minute.

Consider the following scenario: A patient was going into shock following severe trauma. An order was written to give 5 mcg/kg/minute I.V. of dopamine. You go to the emergency cart and find that the dopamine is available in a concentration of 40 mg/ml.

First, make sure that the patient's weight is calculated in kilograms. To convert pounds to kilograms, use the following formula:

$$\frac{\text{known weight}}{\text{weight in kg}} = \frac{2.2 \text{ lb}}{\text{kg}}$$

The patient weighs 200 lb.

$$\frac{200 \text{ lb}}{\text{X kg}} = \frac{2.2 \text{ lb}}{1 \text{ kg}}$$

$$\text{X kg} \times 2.2 \text{ lb} = 200 \text{ lb-kg}$$

$$\text{X kg} = \frac{200 \text{ lb-kg}}{2.2 \text{ lb}}$$

$$\text{X} = 90.9 \text{ kg}$$

Now calculate the dose of drug the patient needs:

$$\frac{\text{patient's weight}}{\text{X mcg/minute}} = \frac{1 \text{ kg}}{\text{ordered dose}}$$

$$\frac{90.9 \text{ kg}}{\text{X mcg/minute}} = \frac{1 \text{ kg}}{5 \text{ mcg/kg}}$$

$$\text{X mcg/minute} \times 1 \text{ kg} = 90.9 \text{ kg} \times 5 \text{ mcg/kg}$$

$$\text{X} = 454.5 \text{ mcg/minute}$$

Because this drug will be delivered by infusion pump, you'll need to determine how much drug is needed per hour by multiplying by 60 minutes/hour.

$$454.5 \text{ mcg/minute} \times 60 \text{ minutes/hour} =$$
$$27,270 \text{ mcg/hour}$$

To prepare the solution for delivery, calculate the concentration to mix. To make all the units the same, convert 40 mg/ml to mcg.

$$1 \text{ mg} = 1,000 \text{ mcg}$$

$$40 \text{ mg} = 40,000 \text{ mcg}$$

Each milliliter of dopamine in solution is equal to 40,000 mcg. The vial contains 5 ml; therefore, the whole vial of solution is added.

You have 250 ml bags of D_5W.

$$\frac{200,000 \text{ mcg}}{250 \text{ ml}} = \text{mcg/ml of solution}$$

$$800 \text{ mcg/ml}$$

Your solution would have 800 mcg/ml. The dose you'll need to deliver would be:

$$\frac{800 \text{ mcg}}{\text{ml}} = \frac{454.5 \text{ mcg/minute}}{\text{X ml/minute}}$$

$$\text{X ml/minute} \times 800 \text{ mcg} = 454.5 \text{ mcg/minute} \times 1 \text{ ml}$$

$$X \text{ ml/minute} = \frac{454.5 \text{ mcg/minute} \times \text{ml}}{800 \text{ mcg}}$$

$$X \text{ ml/minute} = .568$$

To determine the hourly rate so that you can program an infusion system, multiply the ml/minute by 60 minutes/hour:

$$0.568 \text{ ml/minutes} \times 60 \text{ minutes/hour} =$$
$$34.08 \text{ ml/hour}$$

Tips for administering medicated infusions

To avoid errors with medicated infusions, follow these fundamental steps:
- ✦ Calculate the dose.
- ✦ If the infusion isn't premixed, draw up the drug in a syringe, and then add the drug to the I.V. bag.
- ✦ Mix the drug thoroughly.
- ✦ Label the I.V. bag with the drug's name, dosage, time and date it was mixed, and your initials.
- ✦ Hang the solution and administer the drug by infusion pump at the prescribed flow rate or drug dosage.

If you work in an area that uses certain drugs — for example, lidocaine and nitroprusside — all the time, it's sound practice to post a chart to avoid common math errors in an emergent situation. However, when time allows, always double-check the calculations to keep math skills sharp and to offer the best defense against medication errors. Also, never rely on a flow rate calculated by another nurse or the pharmacy. Make it a practice to check all medicated infusions as well as I.V. infusions when assuming care of a patient to avoid continuing an error.

A monitoring tip

Time-taping an I.V. bag helps ensure that a solution is administered at the prescribed rate. It also helps facilitate recording of fluid intake.

To time-tape an I.V. bag, place a strip of adhesive tape from the top to the bottom of the bag, next to the fluid level markings. (This illustration shows a bag time-taped for a rate of 100 ml/hour beginning at 10 a.m.)

0 MARKS THE SPOT

Next to the "0" marking, record the time that you hung the bag. Then, knowing the hourly rate, mark each hour on the tape next to the corresponding fluid marking. At the bottom of the tape, mark the time at which the solution will be completely infused.

INK ALERT

Don't write directly on the bag with a felt tip marker because the ink may seep into the fluid. Some manufacturers provide printed time-tapes for use with their solutions.

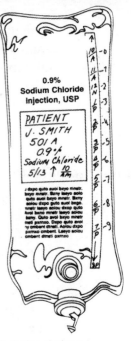

0.9%
Sodium Chloride
Injection, USP

Monitoring the rate

After you've calculated the amount of time and the rate at which an I.V. solution has to infuse, it's important to monitor that solution. If the I.V. is regulated manually, there are factors that can affect the flow rate, such as catheter position in the vein or limb position as well as the helpful patient who feels the need to adjust things on his own. Not getting enough solution as well as inadvertently getting too much may affect the patient. Marking the I.V. bag is an easy way to quickly check if the I.V. is flowing at the calculated rate. (See *A monitoring tip*.)

An I.V. solution is sometimes administered via an electronic pump. Although these devices save time and effort, there's still the possibility of error. The I.V. rate still needs to be calculated correctly and the system needs to be checked to see if it's indeed infusing correctly. An error made in the programming of the pump may actually be more detrimental to the patient because the pump may be more efficient. For example, if the rate is mistakenly set to deliver 500 ml/hour instead of 100 ml/hour, the patient may suffer from fluid overload. Always recheck calculations and settings with any electronic device. Also, check if a medication's infusion rate, such as dopamine, is calculated and set correctly on an electronic pump. The wrong dose can be very damaging to the patient.

✦ Replay: The third right

The third "right" in the common-sense approach to preventing medication errors is to make sure that you administer the right dose. This involves verifying what has been ordered. Many communication errors can occur with respect to a dose in a drug order. Poor handwriting can be misread and misinterpreted. Common problems that can be avoided include improper use of decimal points; run-on words and numbers; misheard numbers, particularly when working with numbers that sound alike, such as 15 and 50; misread abbreviations, such as mistaking "U" (meaning units) for a 0 or 4; and misunderstanding of what's intended in an incomplete order, such as "give one tablet" when tablets may be available in differing doses.

If an order is written in such a way that any part of it is hard to interpret or understand, clarify the entire order.

Always double-check an order when doubt arises about the amount being ordered for a patient: Does it

✦

Checklist for preventing dosage errors

Use this quick checklist to help prevent medication errors related to dosage.
☐ Check the order for clarity:
– Is there a "naked" decimal point (not preceded by a zero) for a dose that's less than one unit?
– Is there a zero following a decimal point that shouldn't be there?
– Do the name of the drug and the dosage ordered run together, or are they clear?
– Are there abbreviations that could be confusing such as "U?"
– Are sound-alike words, such as 14 and 40, clearly understood?
☐ Check to see if the drug dosage ordered makes sense for the patient:
– Is the patient at the extreme for age, weight, or renal or liver function?
☐ Check to see if the dosage to be delivered is accurate and corresponds to the dosage ordered:
– Have mathematical calculations been done correctly?
– Do you need to give more than two or three standard units of the drug?
– Have you checked to make sure a tablet can be cut if a fraction of a dose is needed?
– Does it check correctly when you check your math: dosage being given multiplied by available form dosage equals the dosage ordered?

correspond to the patient's age, weight, and disease state? Post a conversion chart of the formulas for converting an adult dosage to a pediatric dosage. Always double-check mathematical calculations and the formula when using one of these conversion formulas. As a patient advocate and usually the last check before giving a drug, the nurse is in a position to verify that the dose fits the patient.

Calculate the dose being given to ensure that what's available has been properly prepared to match what was ordered. Post a list of conversions in a convenient place so that converting between measurement systems or converting within a system can be double-checked.

Double-check mathematical calculations with another nurse if possible. If this isn't possible, always use the quick check system: the calculated dose multiplied by the available dose should equal the dose that you're about to give. Don't rely on the accuracy of unit-dose or computer systems; errors can happen within these systems, and math skills are readily lost if they aren't used.

Keep math skills sharp and all patients safe. Always verify that what is given converts to what was ordered. And, again, when there's doubt, check it out. (See *Checklist for preventing dosage errors*.)

Chapter

6

The right route

The fourth "right" to consider before administering a drug is whether the drug is being given by the right route. This means assuring that the route that has been ordered is the route that's being used; that it's the appropriate route for this patient; and that the proper administration technique is used.

One of the first things that a nurse learns is proper administration technique for different forms of medication. Instructors check form and technique, and preceptors evaluate procedure. Medication administration soon becomes a comfortable nursing task. However, as with everything that becomes routine, the details of drug administration are often lost over time. Shortcuts may become the norm, and sometimes even the basics are forgotten or overlooked. Although it's difficult to take the time to refresh these skills during a hectic shift or heavy workload, it's an important part of safe medication procedures.

✦ Interpreting the order

Problems involving interpreting the route ordered for drug administration are similar to those encountered when trying to decide what drug or dosage has been ordered. Poor handwriting, poor communication skills, and distractions can lead to a misinterpretation of the intended route.

Problematic abbreviations

Many commonly accepted abbreviations are used in health care. (See *Commonly used medical abbreviations*, pages 214 and 215.) Problems can occur when the abbreviation isn't a standard one or is misinterpreted. An abbreviation can often be misread because of poor handwriting; for example, q.d. is easily understood when typed. However, when written poorly, the period may look like an "i" and the abbreviation may appear to be "qid." A medication given four times per day instead of once can be fatal to the patient.

Specific abbreviations can vary among health care facilities and also among units within facilities. If your practice setting changes, be sure to obtain a list of the abbreviations accepted in your new setting. If such a list isn't available, always question an order in which the abbreviation doesn't make sense or doesn't fit the situation. When in doubt, check it out.

PREVENT IT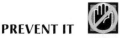

Medication error: *A graduate nurse was undergoing orientation to a new job and was spending 2 weeks on the pediatric floor. A 6-year-old patient developed otitis media and the attending physician ordered: Colymycin drops iii au tid. The secretary transcribing the order interpreted it as: Colymycin drops iii ou tid.*

Because the new nurse wasn't familiar with the abbreviation "ou," she looked it up and found that it meant "both eyes." She administered three drops in each of the child's eyes. The child became hysterical, screaming in pain. The nurse sought help to calm the child, while the charge nurse exam-

(Text continues on page 216.)

Commonly used medical abbreviations

A list of commonly accepted abbreviations used in writing medication orders is shown below.

$\bar{a}$	before		H_2O_2	hydrogen peroxide
$\bar{a}\bar{a}$	of each		h.s.	hour of sleep (bedtime)
a.c.	before meals		I.D.	intradermal
a.d.	right ear		I.M.	intramuscular
a.m.	morning		I.U.	international unit
a.s.	left ear		I.V.	intravenous
a.u.	both ears		K	potassium
b.i.d.	two times per day		KCl	potassium chloride
$\bar{c}$	with		kg	kilogram
cc	cubic centimeter		L	left, liter
cm	centimeter		m	meter
D/C	discontinue; discharge		mcg	microgram
D_5W	dextrose 5% in water		mEq	milliequivalent
Fe	iron		mEq/L	milliequivalent per liter
g	gram		Mg	magnesium
gr	grain		mg	milligram
gtt	drops		ml	milliliter
H_2O	water		MOM	milk of magnesia

Commonly used medical abbreviations *(continued)*

Na	sodium		q	every
NaCl	sodium chloride		q.d.	every day
NG	nasogastric		q4h	every 4 hours
NPO	nothing by mouth		q.h.	every hour
OD	right eye		q.i.d.	four times per day
o.d.	daily		q.o.d.	every other day
OL	left eye		Rx	prescription, treatment, or therapy
OPV	oral polio vaccine		s̄	without
OTC	over-the-counter		S.C.	subcutaneous
OU	both eyes		S.L.	sublingual
P̄	after		stat	immediately
p.c.	after meals		T	tablespoon; temperature
PCA	patient-controlled analgesia		t.i.d.	three times per day
P.O.	by mouth		T.O.	telephone order
pr	per rectum		U	unit
p.r.n.	as needed		USP	United States Pharmacopeia
PT	prothrombin time		V.O.	verbal order
PTT	partial thromboplastin time			

ined the order and the patient's record and realized the error. The attending physician was notified, and he ordered an eye irrigation for the child. The new nurse was totally shocked and needed much support to continue, but the child didn't suffer permanent ill effects from this error.

Prevention: This error was caused by several misinterpretations. First, the secretary misinterpreted the physician's handwriting. Second, although the new nurse was thorough enough to check the order and look up the abbreviation, she didn't check the patient's diagnosis. Had she known that the child had otitis media, she would have questioned the use of eye drops.

Whenever an abbreviation is unfamiliar, check it out completely. Looking it up on a sheet of abbreviations can be a good start, but you should also question the actual order and the use of the drug. Any part of a drug order that raises questions should alert you to the risk of other errors in interpretation. Many facilities recommend that "au" ("both ears") and "ou" ("both eyes") no longer be used because of the possibility of confusion. Writing out the words may take longer, but could save time, effort, and patient problems in the long run.

Some abbreviations are frequently mixed up or misinterpreted and should serve as red flags to potential errors whenever they are used. "IU," which is the usual abbreviation for international units (a system of measurement for some antineoplastic drugs and other particular drugs) has often been misread as "IV."

PREVENT IT

Medication error: Brian, age 26, has had human immunodeficiency virus (HIV) infection for several years and has managed well. He was recently diagnosed with acquired immunodeficiency syndrome (AIDS)-related Kaposi's sarcoma and the physician decided to try treatment with interferon alfa-2a (Roferon-A). An order was written for: 36 million IU daily SC for 10-12 wk. The order was transcribed as: 36 million units IV for 10-12 weeks. The pharmacy sent a vial containing 36 million units.

When the medication nurse went to the room to give the drug, she found that the patient didn't have an intravenous (I.V.) line and was concerned about administering the drug because his veins weren't good. When she asked the physician about having a heparin lock inserted, he questioned the need and the error was discovered. Roferon-A isn't intended for I.V. use, but can be given intramuscularly (I.M.) or subcutaneously (S.C.). The busy secretary who transcribed the order saw the "IU," read it as "IV," and overlooked the "SC."

Prevention: *Whenever a drug is prescribed in IU dosage, a red flag should go up for the person ordering and administering it. There have been several reports involving misinterpretation errors involving IU and I.V. When giving a drug that comes in IU, double-check the order to make sure that the route intended is the route being used.*

Some prescribers write out the Latin "per os" ("by mouth") when ordering an oral drug. Technically, this is accurate. However, "os" is also the accepted abbreviation for left eye. Some errors have occurred when an order written "per os" was actually administered to the left eye. "P.O." is the most commonly accepted abbreviation for oral medications and it should be used, or "by mouth" or "orally" should be written out. When there's a doubt about the meaning of an abbreviation, check it out.

PREVENT IT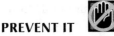

Medication error: *Irene Gordon, a 68-year-old chronic care resident, has a history of chronic cystitis, which often causes her to have very uncomfortable bladder spasms. She was giv-*

en an antibiotic to treat the organisms associated with her current bladder infection and, remembering her bladder spasms, the attending physician also ordered: atropine, 0.4 mg/d per os as long as needed.

The nurse read the order and interpreted the administration route to mean "per left eye." The unit had a stock supply of atropine eye drops and she gave the patient 4 drops in the left eye with her morning medications. When the physician made rounds, he became concerned that one of Irene's pupils was very large. Fearing a neurologic event, he ordered several tests. Before these tests could be scheduled, however, the nursing supervisor reviewed the chart and discovered the problem. Giving atropine via eye drops into only one eye had most likely caused the pupil dilation and wouldn't have helped the urinary bladder spasm. The drug was stopped, and oral tablets were ordered for the patient.

Prevention: This error could have been prevented if the nurse administering the drug had checked to see why the drug was being given. Treating a bladder spasm with eye drops should have raised questions. The use of "per os" to mean "by mouth" is rare, and it's often missing from standard abbreviation lists. The physician in this case should be encouraged to use a more common abbreviation or to write out the route. Following all five "rights" to preventing medication errors would have alerted the nurse to this error before the wrong route was used. Fortunately, the patient suffered no ill effects and the error was discovered before she had to undergo many costly diagnostic tests.

Another frequently misread abbreviation is the one used to mean subcutaneous injection: S.C. This has been confused with SL, which means sublingual. "Sub q," another abbreviation used in some facilities, has been misinterpreted to mean "subcutaneously" and "every." When an order is written for a drug "sub q 2h before meals," it can be interpreted to mean "subcutaneously every 2 hours before meals."

IT'S A FACT

The Institute of Safe Medication Practices (ISMP) has suggested that the abbreviations "S.C." and "sub q" no longer be used. It's recommended that the word "subcutaneous" be written out and never abbreviated.

With health care provider shortages and many sick patients, it's possible that new protocols and procedures will be instituted in the clinical area. Always follow up on any doubts or questions because the nurse administering a drug is responsible for her own actions.

PREVENT IT

Medication error: A surgeon routinely ordered prophylactic heparin for his patients undergoing abdominal surgeries. One such patient was admitted to a medical floor the day before surgery because all of the surgical beds were taken. The staff on this floor wasn't familiar with the surgeon or his standard procedures. He wrote an order for: heparin 5,000 units sub q 2h prior to surgery.

The order was interpreted to mean "heparin, 5,000 units every 2 hours before surgery." Although the medical nurses thought this to be a very high dose of heparin, after discussion they decided that they were probably not familiar with surgical procedures and proceeded to give the heparin every 2 hours through the night. The morning nurse reviewed the orders and became concerned with the large dose of heparin that the patient had received. She reread the order and decided that the surgeon probably meant "subcutaneously 2 hours before surgery." A prothrombin time (PTT) was immediately performed and found to be very prolonged. The surgeon post-

poned the surgery for 1 day until the PTT returned to normal.

Prevention: Fortunately, an alert nurse picked up the error and followed up on the problem before the patient underwent surgery, during which excessive bleeding could have been life-threatening. The reasons for the error were discussed in a staff meeting. The use of "sub q" to mean "subcutaneously" was new to the staff; most had never seen that abbreviation before. The use of "S.C." — the more accepted abbreviation — could have prevented this misinterpretation. The nurses who weren't familiar with the abbreviation but decided to proceed with the order were counseled about a more appropriate method to obtain information. The phrase "When in doubt, check it out" was posted in the staff room.

✦ Availability and appropriateness

Once you've determined the route for a medication, you need to check and make sure that the ordered drug is available for administration by that route. Most nursing drug guides list available forms for each drug. A quick telephone call to the pharmacy can also determine what's available.

You also need to determine if the route ordered is appropriate for the patient. Can the patient swallow a tablet or capsule? Does the patient have good peripheral circulation to allow absorption after an I.M. or S.C. injection? Can the patient manage an inhaled product? You may be in the best position to determine if an ordered drug route is appropriate for a particular patient. Difficulty in swallowing may not be obvious until the patient tries to swallow a tablet. Problems with coordination or eyesight may not be obvious until the patient tries to draw up a syringe, prepares a drug for inhalation, or sprays a sublingual drug into the eyes. Difficulties in reading and interpreting orders may not be apparent until the patient participates in an education program with you.

The pharmacist may sometimes be able to compound a drug so that it can be available in a different form. For example, some antibiotics may not be available in a liquid form, but may be the drug of choice for an infection in a child. Often, the pharmacist will be able to prepare a solution of the drug so that the child can easily take the prescribed drug.

As some diseases progress, patients may develop difficulty swallowing. In the past, some drugs weren't available in a liquid form. To overcome the problem, drug companies manufacturing these drugs provided directions for making these drugs into a liquid for these patients. Many such drugs are now available as oral solutions.

Certain drugs can be made into a suppository form for patients who can't take a drug orally. However, sometimes the drug can't be prepared in a form that's appropriate for the patient. Always check with the pharmacist, who's trained to prepare and dispense drugs, before having the drug of choice changed for a patient. However, remember to never alter the available form of a drug to a different route without first checking with the pharmacist.

PREVENT IT

Medication error: *Nancy Drake, under treatment with imatinib (Gleevec) for chronic myelocytic leukemia (CML), developed a breast nodule that was biopsied and diagnosed as a ductal carcinoma. She was admitted to the surgical unit for a mastectomy. Ms. Drake was concerned about still being able to take her imatinib; she had had a very rough course with her CML until she starting taking this drug. She shared her* *concerns with the graduate nurse who was caring for her pre-operatively.*

The nurse read the order that the patient was to take nothing by mouth after midnight. Worried that Ms. Drake might suffer a relapse or experience other problems if she couldn't take the imatinib, the nurse ground up the tablet and put it into the patient's I.V. solution. She assured the patient that she was getting the drug and that she shouldn't worry. When the nurse manager made her rounds that morning, she noticed particulate matter floating in the I.V. solution and immediately replaced the solution with a fresh bottle. When she questioned the graduate nurse about why she didn't notice the particulate matter in the bottle, the nurse manager discovered how the graduate nurse had administered the drug. Luckily, the particulate matter was too large to actually enter the microdrip chamber and the patient didn't suffer a thrombotic event.

Prevention: *The graduate nurse should have shared the patient's concerns with her supervisor or the patient's physician. Some nurses on the unit weren't surprised or concerned about the administration of oral medications in this manner, raising concerns that this may be a common practice on this particular surgical unit. An aggressive educational series was planned for the unit.*

The nurse shouldn't have altered a drug to make it available by another route. Drugs are prepared in specific mediums or binders for particular routes of administration. Most drugs can't be transformed to a different route just by making them physically able to be given by that route. If a drug is ordered to be given by a route that won't work for the patient, check it out. Is another form of the drug available? Can the pharmacist prepare the drug to be given by a different route? Should a different drug be ordered for this patient at this time?

✦ Giving oral medications

Oral drugs are the most frequently used drugs because they're less expensive, more convenient, and usually the safest route for delivering drugs. Oral medications may come in tablets or capsules, powders or granules, liquids (which may be suspensions, elixirs, or syrups), or sprays (such as nitroglycerin). Some medications need to be mixed in applesauce or a specific juice; others can't be mixed with food. Certain medications can be crushed, cut, or chewed; others must be swallowed whole. Giving an oral medication isn't as simple as handing the patient a tablet and a glass of water; there are other considerations to assess before administering an oral drug.

Crushing tablets

If a patient has problems swallowing, check to make sure that the prescribed drug can be crushed. Many drugs used today can't be crushed, cut, or chewed. If the drug can be crushed, use a mortar and pestle to crush it, and then make sure that all the remnants of the drug are put into the applesauce or other vehicle being used to deliver the drug. Then it's very important to clean the mortar and pestle so that the next patient whose drug is crushed in it isn't exposed to the previous drug.

The use of unit-dose packaging can make crushing a drug an easier task. Some unit-dose packages can be placed in the mortar and the drug crushed and then emptied out of the package into the vehicle.

PREVENT IT

Medication error: A traveling nurse was placed in a chronic care facility for a 2-week rotation. The patients in the facility were elderly and many had Alzheimer's disease or similar neurologic disorders that made swallowing difficult. To facilitate her schedule for delivering medications, the nurse took all of a patient's medications and crushed them when she arrived at the room, and gave the crushed remnants in applesauce. The nurse repeated this for all patients and all drugs. When questioned by a patient's visitor about giving crushed tablets when the patient didn't seem to have trouble swallowing in the past, the nurse responded that it was facility procedure.

Mr. Jones was admitted to the facility following an emergency appendectomy and was still receiving some medication for pain. He had orders for 2 more days of sustained-release oxycodone (Oxycontin). The nurse crushed the oxycodone with the rest of his medications and gave them to him in applesauce. About 30 minutes after giving him the medications, the nurse was called to the room by a concerned visitor who noted that Mr. Jones had become very flushed and was agitated and talking incoherently. His blood pressure was very low and his respiratory rate was only 10 breaths/minute.

The nurse called for help to provide supportive care. An I.V. line was started, and the patient was closely monitored for 3 hours before his vital signs started to normalize. Reviewing the day's events in rounds that evening, the nurses found nothing unusual and no changes in Mr. Jones' regimen. A nurse mentioned that oxycodone had been on a popular news program that day with stories of people cutting the tablet to get high from the concentrated opioid effects that occur when the tablet's coating is broken and all of the sustained-release drug is absorbed at the same time. When the traveling nurse inquired whether this could happen if the drug was crushed, the error was discovered. The nurse said that she hadn't been taught that certain drugs can't be crushed, and had felt that all patients in the facility would be served better if they got their oral drugs in crushed form.

Prevention: Although the patient survived, this medication error could have had a very different result. Drugs that can't be cut, crushed, or chewed have increased markedly *since the invention of slow-release forms for drugs. A list of drugs that can't be altered in this way should be posted in the medication room, on the medication cart, or at the nurses' station when such drugs are used in a unit. Nurses who learned to give medications when crushing drugs wasn't considered a problem should attend a refresher course on new delivery systems and the problems that arise when such drugs are altered. If a drug appears new to you or isn't scored so it appears that it shouldn't be cut, check it out.*

A technical aspect of crushing drugs that often gets lost over time is the cleaning of the mortar and pestle after each use. If these utensils aren't cleaned after use, the next drug crushed with these utensils may be mixed with remnants of the previous drug and may cause harm to the patient.

PREVENT IT

Medication error: *The medication nurse on the rehabilitation unit was pulled from the holding unit where patients wait for placement in other facilities. The pace of the rehabilitation unit was much more hectic than she was used to; however, there was a shortage of nurses and she was desperately needed to pass out medications. Many patients on the rehabilitation unit were recovering from strokes or head injuries, and many had to have their medications crushed for oral use. The medication cart had a mortar and pestle and the nurse began carefully checking, crushing, and administering the medications and then cleaning the mortar and pestle with the paper towels on the cart. As the day progressed and the pace of activity increased, the nurse became increasingly stressed and the process and patients became somewhat blurred. Toward the end of the shift, a patient experienced difficulty breathing, became flushed and anxious, and proceeded to*

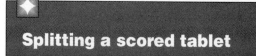

Splitting a scored tablet

If a tablet is scored, use a cutting device to break the tablet cleanly. Place the tablet into the device so the score mark lines up with the blade. Close the lid of the cutting device to force the blade through the tablet, as shown below.

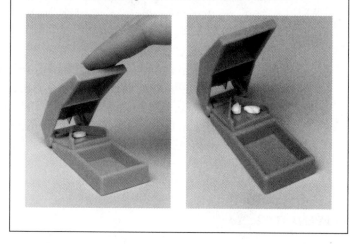

have an anaphylactic reaction that required emergency support.

Once the patient was rescued from the reaction and stabilized, the staff began to investigate the cause of his reaction. There was nothing different about medications, food, or exposures to airborne allergens that they could discover. The patient had a severe allergy to penicillin with anaphylaxis noted on the chart. However, penicillin wasn't given to the patient. The staff checked to see if another patient in the room had been given penicillin thinking, perhaps, a mix-up may have occurred. That, too, wasn't found to be the case. The staff tracked down two patients who were receiving penicillin. One of those patients and the patient who had the anaphylactic reaction had to have their medications crushed. The patient receiving penicillin was the last patient to have his medication crushed before this patient who had the reaction was given his drug. Although the stressed medication nurse believed that she had been careful to clean the utensils each time she gave the medications, she admitted that she was overwhelmed by the afternoon and may have slipped up. It was determined that the patient had reacted to the remnants of the penicillin that remained on the pestle and in the mortar.

Prevention: This error could have been prevented if the nurse had been able to maintain her routine of cleaning the mortar and pestle after each use. It's easy to understand how she became overwhelmed and how this mistake occurred. Unfortunately, it's also easy to imagine a similar error happening on any busy unit. This incident was used as a reminder to the staff of the potential for serious consequences when shortcuts are taken with medication administration. Educational review sessions were held to remind nurses of the importance of cleaning the mortar and pestle between each use.

Splitting tablets

Splitting tablets can be a tricky business because not all tablets and pills are scored. If a tablet is scored, use a cutting device to break the tablet cleanly. (See *Splitting a scored tablet.*) However, if a cutting device isn't available, place the tablet in a paper towel and grip the tablet on either side of the score mark to break it. If the tablet isn't scored, it shouldn't be split because it may not break easily and the patient then wouldn't be receiving the prescribed dose of the drug.

Problems with swallowing

When giving a patient an oral medication, make sure that the patient has enough water to swallow it. Some tablets and capsules are large and may become lodged in the esophagus. Certain oral drugs that come as powders or granules need fluid to wash them down into the stomach. Also, make sure that the patient is sitting upright. Don't expect a patient to safely swallow an oral medication from a reclining position — it's possible for him to aspirate the drug.

PREVENT IT

Medication error: A student nurse was assigned to take care of two patients. One patient was to undergo a thyroidectomy that morning and the other, Mrs. Weber, was being prepared for diagnostic tests. The student nurse was hurrying to prepare everything for the surgical patient before he left for surgery. While she was passing medications to Mrs. Weber, the transporter came for the surgical patient. The student gave Mrs. Weber her medications, including Metamucil, and saw that her bedside pitcher had little water. Feeling rushed, the student had Mrs. Weber take her other medications with as little water as possible and then the Metamucil followed by the remaining sip of water. The student rushed out to help transport the surgical patient.

Within 10 minutes, Mrs. Weber became very anxious, gasping for breath, and complaining of severe chest pressure. She was given a glass of water. However, the symptoms continued to worsen, her blood pressure fell, and she lost consciousness. The emergency response team worked on the patient and, eventually, it was determined that Mrs. Weber had ruptured her esophagus. She was rushed to surgery and survived. In rounds following the emergency procedure, it was explained that the Metamucil — which is a bulk laxative that works by pulling in fluid and expanding — had become lodged in her esophagus, where it started to expand. Giving her the glass of water allowed the bulk to expand dramatically and it ruptured her esophagus.

Prevention: The student nurse, who had looked up all the medications her patients were taking, wasn't really familiar with the way the medications worked. She could recite their *actions, but didn't seem to be able to apply those actions to what transpired with the patient. She learned a valuable lesson: Never give an oral medication to a patient without enough water to ensure that it's completely swallowed. It may take a little time to fill a water pitcher or get a patient a glass of water, but it could save time and patient problems in the long run.*

Pouring liquid medications

When giving a liquid medication, remember that it needs to be measured carefully if it isn't supplied in a unit-dose package. Most facilities use plastic, graduated medicine cups for this purpose. When reading the graduations, it's important to remember to use the bottom of the meniscus as the measuring indicator. When reading the measure on the cup, make sure that it's at eye level. If this detail seems unimportant, pour water into a glass measuring cup and read the volume while standing above the cup; now bend over and read the volume at eye level. It will be quite different. (See *Measuring liquid drugs,* page 230.)

Also remember that a spoonful of medicine should be measured out with the correct device. Don't use a plastic spoon. Use the graduated medicine cup already mentioned; it also has teaspoon and tablespoon indications on it.

A consideration with liquid medication is the amount the patient needs to take. For certain medications, such as GO-LYTELY (a drug given for bowel preparation), the patient needs to ingest a large amount (4 L total). Because it's impossible to remain with the patient while he drinks such medications, use good judgment about trusting the patient to drink the entire amount. Repeatedly check on the patient to monitor his progress with drinking the solution. If the

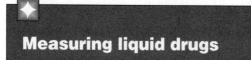

Measuring liquid drugs

To measure a liquid drug accurately, hold the graduated medication cup at eye level. Use your thumbnail to mark the correct dose level on the cup.

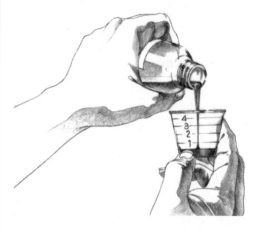

Hold the bottle with the label side up so the liquid flows from the opposite side of the label; this way, the liquid won't stain or obscure the label if it runs down the bottle.

Pour the liquid into the cup until the bottom of the meniscus reaches the correct dose amount. Then set the cup down and read the bottom of the meniscus again — still at eye level — to double-check your accuracy. If you've poured too much, discard the excess rather than pouring it back into the bottle. Remove any drips from the lip of the bottle using a damp paper towel. Then clean the sides of the bottle if necessary.

patient is untrustworthy, or unable to remember to keep drinking the solution, give him the medication in small amounts and stay with him while he drinks it. Although this is time-consuming, it may be necessary to ensure that the patient takes the entire medication.

Squirting medications

Giving oral medications to infants and children can be challenging. Syringe-like delivery devices or droppers are often used to get medication into a child's mouth. The child's position is an important factor. Be sure to hold the child at least at a 45-degree angle to help facilitate swallowing and prevent aspiration, as shown below. Insert the liquid into the pocket between the child's cheek and gum; this should prevent the child from spitting it out directly.

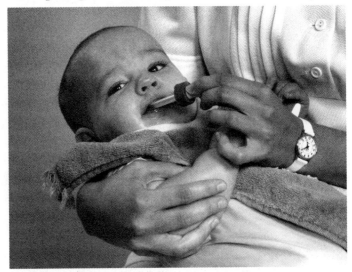

These are important points to teach parents who will give a child medication at home. It's also critical to make sure that the parents understand that the syringe-type delivery systems that are used for oral medications aren't the same as hypodermic syringes.

IT'S A FACT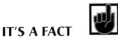

Hypodermic syringes are used to draw up an exact amount of a liquid medication and then to instill it directly into a child's mouth or throat; this method ensures that the correct dose is drawn up and eliminates loss through spilling or the child's refusal to take the drug. Unfortunately, medications can actually be drawn into some syringes while the syringe cap is still in place. Because the caps are often transparent, many parents may not be aware of their existence. The cap can be propelled into the child's throat when the drug is administered. The ISMP warns all parents never to use a hypodermic syringe to administer oral medication.

When administering liquid medicine, be sure to use measuring spoons or specially designed oral syringes. The oral syringe caps are designed to resist the pressure of a plunger, which could send them off during drug administration. These caps are easy to remove to draw up the drug and are usually brightly colored — a visible reminder to remove them. Health care providers involved in patient education should be acutely aware of this potential problem and should encourage parents to use only the oral syringes if they choose to use this method of drug administration.

Oral absorption

Some drugs aren't meant to be swallowed, but are delivered through the mucous membrane of the mouth. This route can provide a faster absorption and is commonly the route of choice when a rapid drug effect is required — for example, when giving drugs to treat an angina attack.

Sublingual administration

Some drugs are designed to be taken sublingually — that is, under the tongue. Patients often prefer to do this themselves. It's important, however, to check for ulcerations or abrasions under the tongue, which could alter absorption or cause pain. Also, the patient should alternate dose placement—the left side of the tongue for one dose, the right side for the next.

Before the patient takes a sublingual tablet, suggest that he drink a sip of water; moistening the mucous membrane will help the drug dissolve more easily. Instruct the patient to place the tablet under his tongue, as shown below, close his mouth, and hold the tablet in place until it dissolves.

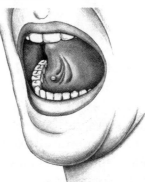

Caution the patient not to swallow the tablet because its effectiveness would be lost. If a patient can't open his mouth or move his tongue, place the sublingual tablet by moving the tongue to one side using a tongue depressor, or by sliding the tablet through a straw to the spot under the tongue.

Buccal administration
Certain drugs are designed to be administered buccally—that is, between the teeth and gums as shown at top of next page. These medications should be held in place until they dissolve and shouldn't be swallowed. Patients often prefer to place the tablet themselves. It's important, however, to assess the patient's mouth and gums first to make sure he doesn't have any ulcerations or abrasions. Buccal tablets should also be dissolved on alternate sides with each dose to avoid excessive irritation.

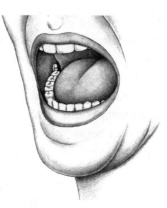

Translingual administration

Some drugs are designed to be administered translin-
gually — that is, applied to the top of the tongue, usually as a spray. Nitroglycerin, used to treat angina attacks, is now available in a translingual spray. In this
form, nitroglycerin is more stable when stored than
sublingual nitroglycerin. Teach the patient how to administer this spray at home, as shown below, if it's intended to treat angina attacks.

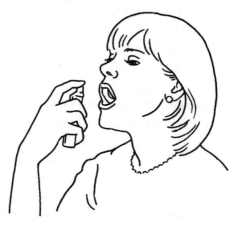

Problems occur when the canister isn't held upright
or is held too far away from the mouth. There have
been many reports of patients who have inadvertently
sprayed the drug into their eyes. Remind the patient
not to breathe in while spraying the drug to avoid inhaling the drug, and not to rinse out his mouth after

using the drug, even if he experiences a bad taste. Nitroglycerin needs to stay in contact with the mucous membranes as long as possible. As with other drugs delivered onto the oral mucous membranes, it's very important to periodically assess the mouth for ulcerations or abrasions that could interfere with the drug's effectiveness.

✦ Giving gastric medications

Some patients receive their oral medications through nasogastric (NG) tubes or gastrostomy tubes. Administering medication using this route still requires checking the five "rights," and then using the correct technique

Nasogastric tube

Always make sure that the patient is in a semi-Fowler's position before administering the drug. Remove the clamp from the nasogastric (NG) tube and check to make sure that the tube is in the right place. Do this by inserting about 10 ml of air into the tube and auscultating for the gurgling sound of the air in the stomach area, as shown below.

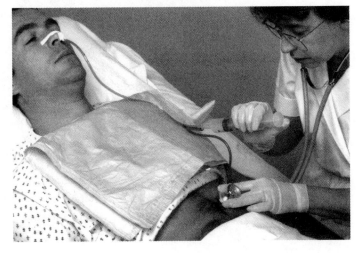

Irrigate the tube with 30 ml of water to remove excess feeding or other backup material. Insert the syringe snugly and slowly pour in the drug. Raise the syringe to increase the flow of the drug; lower the syringe to slow the flow. After the drug has gone in, flush the remaining drug into the stomach with 30 to 50 ml of water. Clamp the tube and leave the patient in the semi-Fowler's position for about 30 minutes. *Don't* reattach suction if the patient has been on continuous suction; instead, return after about 1 hour and reattach the suction.

PREVENT IT

Medication error: James, recovering from a severe automobile accident and experiencing seizures, had an NG tube placed to deliver feedings and prevent aspiration from swallowing. The nurse who gave him his morning medications was unfamiliar with delivering medications by this route. She looked up the process in the procedure manual and carefully crushed his medications, elevated his head, disconnected the suction, flushed the tube, slowly delivered the medications, and flushed the tube again. As she removed the syringe from the tube, she didn't know what to do with the end of the tube and decided that it should be reattached to the original tubing.

Two hours later, James' mother came to the desk to report that he was twitching again and she was afraid he was about to have more seizures. Supportive measures were taken and James was given an I.V. dose of his anticonvulsant medication. When cleaning out the drainage container, the night nurse noticed that the drainage didn't look like it usually did and left a note asking if James had been given something different or if the tube could be out of place. The day shift nurse who was taking care of James noticed that when the medication nurse gave his medications, she immediately reattached the tube to the suction and a lot of fluid drained out. Questioning the medication nurse, it was discovered that the day before, and again that day, the nurse had given James his medication and then it was immediately suctioned out because the nurse didn't know that suctioning should be discontinued for 1 hour after drug administration.

Prevention: The medication nurse had looked up the procedure and felt that she had followed it well. It would have been better if she had been shown how to deliver medication via an NG tube. It may be a good idea for staff development nurses to follow the procedures written in a book to see where they might be confusing or incomplete. The nurse administering a medication by a new or different route should feel free to ask for assistance or a demonstration. The nurse administering a drug is responsible for its proper delivery.

Gastrostomy tube

Gastrostomy tubes are used similarly to NG tubes. Stop feedings for about 1 hour after drugs are administered. The actual procedure varies depending on the pump being used. The drug should flow into the stomach slowly and the tube flushed afterward. Dressing care should be done at the same time if needed. (See *Giving drugs through a gastrostomy tube,* page 238.)

✦ Giving ophthalmic and otic medications

Drugs applied directly to the eye or into the ear are used for diagnostic purposes or to treat infections or diseases associated with these areas without some of the systemic adverse effects associated with oral or parenteral drugs. However, these drugs may be absorbed systemically in some situations. All of the cautions and contraindications associated with systemic use should be considered before using these drugs.

Giving drugs through a gastrostomy tube

Medications are sometimes given through a gastrostomy tube. Make sure the patient is in a semi-Fowler's position before giving the drug by this route. Remove the piston from the catheter-tipped syringe and insert the catheter into the gastrostomy tube. Instill 30 ml of water into the syringe to flush the feeding solution through the tube and into the patient's stomach. This allows you to check the tube's patency and to clear the tube before giving a drug through it.

Slowly pour up to 30 ml of the drug at a time into the syringe, as shown below. Allow the drug to flow slowly through the tube, adding more drug as the syringe empties but before it drains completely. After giving the full dose, flush the tube with 30 ml water. Carefully remove the syringe from the tube and tighten the clamp or replug the opening of the tube.

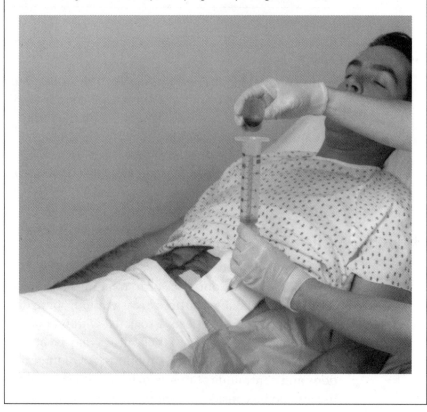

Ophthalmic drugs

Drugs applied directly to the eye are usually given as drops or ointments. An ocular disk may also be used. Review the specifics for administering ophthalmic medication periodically because the details are often lost over time.

Before applying an eye medication, wash your hands thoroughly. Be sure to clean around the eye to remove any discharge or crusted secretions. To clean the eye, moisten sterile cotton balls or gauze pads with warm water or normal saline solution to remove crusted secretions or debris. Wipe the eye gently, moving from the inner canthus to the outer canthus, as shown below. Use a fresh sterile cotton ball or gauze for each stroke.

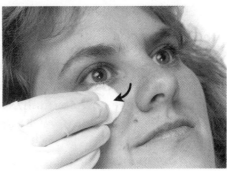

Eyedrops

Eyedrops may be used for diagnostic purposes, as well as to anesthetize, lubricate, and treat certain disorders. Be sure you understand why the drug is being given before you administer it.

When applying drops, don't touch the eyedropper to the patient's eye or any other surface. Instruct the patient to tilt his head backward. Grasp the lower eyelid and pull it gently away from the eyeball, as shown at top of next page. Instill the prescribed number of drops into the conjunctival pouch formed by the eyelid and release the lid slowly. Have the patient close the eye and look downward while applying gentle pressure to the inner corner of the eye for 3 to 5 minutes. Advise him not to rub the eye. Don't rinse the eyedropper, but replace it in the bottle. If a patient isn't getting the desired effect from an ophthalmic medication, review the administration technique carefully.

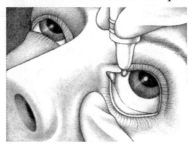

Eye ointment

An ointment formulation keeps medication in contact with the treatment area longer than drops. Warm the ointment in your hands for several minutes before administration. Wash your hands thoroughly and have the patient lie down or tilt his head back. Gently pull out the patient's lower eyelid and apply the ointment to the inside of the lower lid, as shown below. Be careful not to touch the tube to the eye or any other surface. Have the patient close his eyes for 1 to 2 minutes and roll his eyes in all directions to disperse the drug. Carefully wipe off any ointment remaining around the eye. If a patient doesn't roll his eyes, the drug won't be dispersed and its effectiveness may be lost.

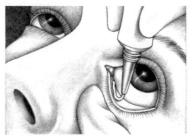

Ocular disk

A medicated ocular disk is a small, flexible, oval wafer that contains medication situated between two soft outer layers. It may be left in place up to 1 week. (See *Using an eye medication disk*, pages 242 and 243.)

Otic drugs

Eardrops are often used to treat infections, to decrease pain associated with ear infections, to reduce inflammation, or to loosen cerumen. Double-check that the medication is meant to be an otic preparation. Warm the solution before administration; cold solutions in the ear can cause vertigo, pain, and even nausea.

Wash your hands thoroughly. Inspect the ear canal to ensure that there are no obstructions to drug delivery. Also, check periodically that the patient has an intact eardrum; otic medications shouldn't be used when an eardrum is perforated unless sterile technique is used, and then only with certain medications.

Position the patient properly for the medication to be most effective, as shown below for an adult and at top of page 244 for a child. Hold the ear auricle in position as you release the eardrops into the ear canal; continue holding the lobe until the drop disappears down the ear canal.

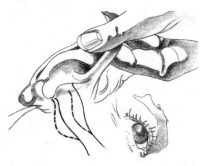

(Text continues on page 244.)

Using an eye medication disk

Small and flexible, an oval eye medication disk consists of three layers: two soft outer layers and a middle layer that contains the medication. Floating between the eyelids and the sclera, the disk stays in the eye while the patient sleeps and even during swimming and athletic activities. The disk frees the patient from having to remember to instill his eyedrops. Once the disk is in place, ocular fluid moistens it, releasing the medication. Eye moisture or contact lenses don't adversely affect the disk. The disk can release medication for up to 1 week before needing replacement. Pilocarpine, for example, can be administered this way to treat glaucoma.

Contraindications include conjunctivitis, keratitis, retinal detachment, and any condition in which constriction of the pupil should be avoided.

TO INSERT AN EYE MEDICATION DISK

Arrange to insert the disk before the patient goes to bed. *This minimizes the blurring that usually occurs immediately after disk insertion.*

✦ Wash your hands and put on gloves.
✦ Press your fingertip against the oval disk so that it lies lengthwise across your fingertip. It should stick to your finger. Lift the disk out of its packet.
✦ Gently pull the patient's lower eyelid away from the eye and place the disk in the conjunctival sac, as shown below. It should lie horizontally, not vertically. The disk will adhere to the eye naturally.

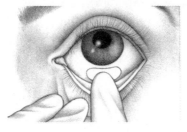

✦ Pull the lower eyelid out, up, and over the disk. Tell the patient to blink several times. If the disk is still visible, pull the lower lid out and over the disk again. Tell the patient that once the disk is in place, he can adjust its position by *gently* pressing his finger against his closed lid. Caution him against rubbing his eye or moving the disk across the cornea.
✦ If the disk falls out, wash your hands, rinse the disk in cool water, and

Using an eye medication disk *(continued)*

reinsert it. If the disk appears bent, replace it.

✦ If both of the patient's eyes are being treated with medication disks, replace both disks at the same time so that both eyes receive medication at the same rate.

✦ If the disk repeatedly slips out of position, reinsert it under the upper eyelid. To do this, gently lift and evert the upper eyelid and insert the disk in the conjunctival sac. Then gently pull the lid back into position, and tell the patient to blink several times. Again, the patient may press gently on the closed eyelid to reposition the disk. The more the patient uses the disk, the easier it should be for him to retain it. If he can't retain it, notify the physician.

✦ If the patient will continue therapy with an eye medication disk after discharge, teach him how to insert and remove it himself. To check his mastery of these skills, have him demonstrate insertion and removal techniques.

✦ Also, teach the patient about possible adverse reactions. Foreign-body sensation in the eye, mild tearing or redness, increased mucous discharge, eyelid redness, and itchiness can occur with the use of disks. Blurred vision, stinging, swelling, and headaches can occur with pilocarpine specifically. Mild symptoms are common but should subside within the first 6 weeks of use. Tell the patient to report persistent or severe symptoms to his physician.

TO REMOVE AN EYE MEDICATION DISK

✦ You can remove an eye medication disk with one or two fingers. To use one finger, put on gloves and evert the lower eyelid to expose the disk. Then use the forefinger of your other hand to slide the disk onto the lid and out of the patient's eye. To use two fingers, evert the lower lid with one hand to expose the disk. Then pinch the disk with the thumb and forefinger of your other hand and remove it from the eye.

✦ If the disk is located in the upper eyelid, apply long circular strokes to the patient's closed eyelid with your finger until you can see the disk in the corner of the patient's eye. Once the disk is visible, place your finger directly on the disk and move it to the lower sclera. Then remove it as you would a disk located in the lower lid.

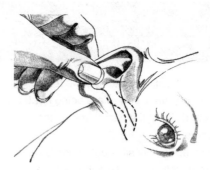

Release the ear and have the patient remain on his side for 5 to 10 minutes to keep the drug in the ear canal. Be gentle to avoid damage to the eardrum when administering these drugs.

PREVENT IT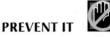

Medication error: *Peter Mullin, age 4, had repeated ear infections and experienced severe pain with each infection. His pediatrician ordered Cortisporin Otic — a combination antibiotic, steroid drug — for his latest infection. His mother was instructed to apply 2 to 3 drops in the affected ear three to four times daily. After 2 days, the mother called the pediatrician's office to report that Peter wasn't better and she had to fight with him to administer the drops. She wanted another treatment for the child. The nurse discussed the use of the drops with her and found that the mother hadn't paid attention to the instructions she was given before she left the office with the prescription. Peter had been upset and uncooperative that day, and she had just wanted to leave. At home, she hadn't been using the drops correctly, but had tried to squirt them into his ear while he was running away.*

The mother was asked to bring Peter in for an evaluation. With Peter there, the nurse administered the drops appropriately and he reported that the pain lessened within a few minutes. The proper technique was reviewed with the mother and she was asked to bring Peter back in 1 week for further evaluation.

Prevention: Otic solution doesn't work when it isn't administered correctly. The staff should have been aware of the situation and the mother's inability to listen or learn while she was in the office. The pharmacist should have explained the administration technique when the mother picked up the drug, although she may have gone to pick it up with the upset Peter in tow. The staff made a note to call the mother the next day, to ask her to review the procedure, and to check on how things were going. It's a good policy to call parents routinely when they're given a new drug, procedure, or regimen for their child's care to make sure that your instructions were heard and understood.

✦ Giving nasal drugs

Sometimes drugs are administered nasally to produce local effects on the nasal mucosa or to anesthetize the nasal passages for diagnostic procedures. Nasal drugs may be administered by drops, spray, or an aerosol device. Before administering a drug by the nasal route, encourage the patient to blow his nose to clear the nasal passages. Advise the patient to breathe through his mouth during drug administration to facilitate delivery of the drug to the correct area and to avoid aspiration of the drug into the lungs.

Periodically, inspect the nasal mucosa for abrasions or lesions that could alter drug absorption. Patients with nasal abrasions are usually not candidates for drugs administered nasally.

Nasal drops

Nasal drops are intended to reach areas of the sinuses that might not be reached by the usual drug delivery routes. The affected sinuses determine the positioning of the patient for drug administration. (See *Positioning the patient for nose drop instillation*.)

Place the dropper about ⅓" (0.8 cm) inside the nares and insert the number of drops ordered. To prevent contamination, don't touch the sides of the nostrils. Instruct the patient to remain in this position for about 5 minutes to allow the drug to flow into the sinuses. Have someone stay with the patient during this 5-minute period to support his head and to ensure his safety.

Nasal spray

Nasal sprays are often used to treat nasal congestion and rhinitis and are usually used for over-the-counter (OTC) drugs designed for allergy or cold symptoms. Instruct the patient to sit upright and press a finger over one nostril to close it. Then, with the spray bottle held upright, have him place the tip of the bottle about ½" (1.5 cm) into his open nostril. A firm squeeze should deliver the drug to the target nasal area.

Caution the patient not to use excessive force to deliver the drug; this could propel the drug into the sinuses and cause additional problems. Don't assume that the patient knows how to use a nasal spray. If he'll be using the nasal spray at home, review the administration procedure with him.

Nasal aerosol

Some nasal delivery devices are designed to propel very fine particles into the nasal passages using a metered drug delivery system such as Turbinaire. Instruct the patient who's using one of these devices to sit upright with his head tilted back. Place the medication cartridge into the plastic nasal adapter and shake well.

Positioning the patient for nose drop instillation

To reach the ethmoid and sphenoid sinuses, have the patient lie on her back with her neck hyperextended and her head tilted back over the edge of the bed. Support her head with one hand to prevent neck strain.

To reach the maxillary and frontal sinuses, have the patient lie on her back with her head toward the affected side and hanging slightly over the edge of the bed. Ask her to rotate her head laterally after hyperextension, and support her head with one hand to prevent neck strain.

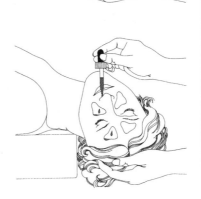

To administer drops to relieve ordinary nasal congestion, help the patient to a reclining or supine position with her head tilted slightly toward the affected side. Aim the dropper upward, toward the patient's eye, rather than downward, toward her ear.

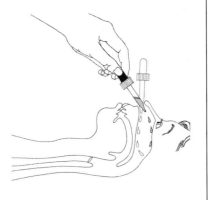

Remove the protective cap from the applicator tip and place this tip inside the patient's nostril. Firmly press once on the cartridge and then release. Ask the patient to inhale or hold his breath for a few seconds. Remove and recap the applicator tip. Ask the patient to exhale, keeping the head tilted back, and to avoid blowing his nose for at least 2 minutes.

PREVENT IT

Medication error: *John Glover, a 23-year-old graduate student, was suffering from seasonal rhinitis. The University Health Service physician decided to try him on Pulmicort (budesonide), a corticosteroid that's effective in relieving the symptoms of seasonal rhinitis. When he picked up his prescription, the pharmacy technician asked if he was familiar with the nasal delivery system and he responded that he could figure it out. At home, he glanced at the directions in the package and tried to follow them, but found the procedure awkward and difficult. That night he saw someone using an inhaler for exercise-induced asthma on television and decided that he should be placing the nasal applicator in his mouth with his head upright and compressing the cartridge into his mouth. The procedure was easier, but he had a terrible taste in his mouth and didn't seem to be getting any benefit from the drug.*

At a follow-up visit, Mr. Glover related his difficulty and asked the nurse to demonstrate how to administer the drug. The nurse explained the difference between an inhaler and the nasal aerosol delivery system. She showed John how to administer the drug and then asked him to repeat the procedure. At his next follow-up visit, John was much improved.

Prevention: *This patient wasted much of his expensive prescription and continued to suffer needlessly because he didn't administer the drug correctly. Patient education is paramount when a patient receives a new drug, a different* *administration technique, or a new drug regimen. Periodically review the procedure with patients who have been using the nasal aerosol administration route. Simple steps—such as shaking the canister, holding one's breath for a few seconds, or not blowing one's nose for several minutes—can become easily forgotten. Always check the nasal mucosa periodically to assess for inflammation, erosion, or irritation that could interfere with drug absorption.*

✦ Giving inhaled drugs

Sometimes it's desirable to deliver drugs directly to the mucosa of the lungs to achieve a rapid reaction and avoid systemic effects associated with these drugs. Many drugs administered by this route are used to treat asthma, bronchitis, or other obstructive pulmonary disorders. Drugs can be delivered for inhalation using an inhaler, a nebulizer or, sometimes, an intermittent positive-pressure breathing (IPPB) device. (See *Types of handheld inhalers,* page 250.)

Inhalers

Inhaler devices allow a canister of drug to be inserted into a dose-metered device that will deliver a measured amount of the drug when the patient compresses the canister. Although an inhaler resembles the device used to deliver nasal aerosol drugs, it has a mouthpiece instead of a nasal tip. A spacer is often used to hold the dose of the drug for delivery while the patient inhales. The spacer is placed in the mouth and is a more exact method of delivering the drug if the patient is somewhat uncoordinated or has trouble inhaling and compressing at the same time.

First, have the patient shake the canister. Then ask him to exhale. Instruct him to place his lips around the

Types of handheld inhalers

Handheld inhalers use air under pressure to produce a mist containing tiny droplets of medication. Drugs delivered in this form (such as mucolytics and bronchodilators) can travel deep into the lungs.

Metered-dose inhaler	Turbo-inhaler with capsules	Nasal inhaler	Inhaler with built-in spacer

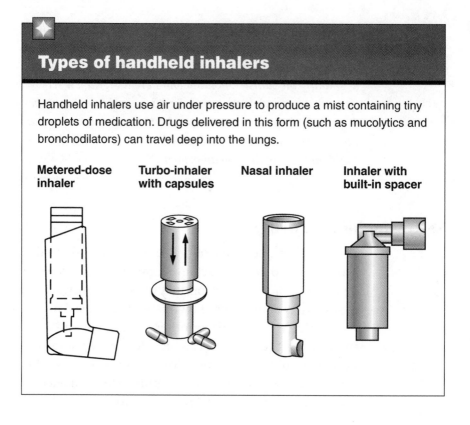

spacer mouthpiece, or hold the device without a spacer 1″ (2.5 cm) from his open mouth; then tell him to compress the canister while inhaling. Advise the patient to hold his breath as long as possible, then exhale through pursed lips. Stress the importance of rinsing his mouth to get rid of excess drug and washing the spacer after use to prevent buildup of drug and by-products.

A special delivery device is used to administer powder for inhalation. Because each device is slightly unique, instruct the patient on how to use the device associated with the drug ordered. When powder for inhalation is used, don't shake the canister before use. Tell the patient to exhale before the inhaler is brought near the mouth; these devices are activated when the

✦ Using an inhaler

Different delivery systems are used to take inhaled medications. The following illustrations depict some different methods.

Oral inhaler

InspirEase system

Oral inhaler with a holding chamber

Aerochamber system

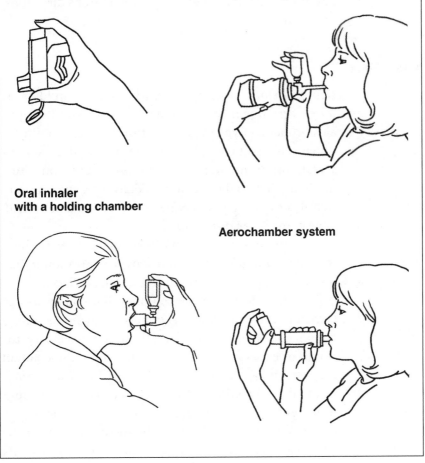

patient inserts the mouthpiece and then forcefully inhales. Encourage the patient to rinse his mouth after each use of this inhaler. (See *Using an inhaler*.)

Patients who use inhalers may use them for years, and the procedure becomes routine for them. To ensure continued correct administration procedure, periodically watch your patient use the inhaler. A patient may forget to exhale before use, to hold his breath after use, or to rinse out his mouth. Because some inhalers work differently, if a patient is given a different brand of inhaler, review the manufacturer's directions with him.

Nebulizers

Nebulizers use compressed air to change a liquid drug into a very fine mist for inhalation. Nebulizer therapy aids bronchial hygiene by restoring and maintaining mucous blanket continuity; hydrating dried, retained secretions; promoting expectoration of secretions; humidifying inspired oxygen; and delivering medications. Nebulizer treatments may be delivered via a handheld device, mask, or respirator.

If a patient is using a handheld device or mask, he should sit upright or in a semi-Fowler's position to improve delivery of the drug into the lungs. Place the correct drug dosage in the chamber that will be attached to the compressed gas source. Encourage the patient to take slow, deep breaths and, if necessary, to cough or expectorate during the treatment. If a patient is noncompliant with the delivery method (for example, fails to keep the mouthpiece in place or keeps removing the mask), monitor his treatment so he receives the complete effects of the medication. After the drug has been delivered, advise the patient to rinse his mouth and gargle, if possible, to remove excess drug.

Patients on respirators are often unaware of receiving medication. The drug is inserted into a cup on the respirator, and the nebulizer is controlled by programming the respirator, which delivers the drug throughout the lungs.

PREVENT IT

Medication error: *Walter Smith, age 81, was admitted to the hospital with pneumonia and a history of chronic obstructive pulmonary disease (COPD) and diabetes. He was started on I.V. antibiotics and albuterol by nebulization to keep his airways open and to prevent bronchospasm. His elderly wife was with him during the day and commented to the attending physician that the nurse would come in, put the drug in the nebulizer, put a mask on the patient, and leave. An hour later, the wife would remove the mask because it was cutting into the patient's face. When the patient had been receiving nebulization treatments at home, the visiting nurse would sit him upright, listen to his lungs, and encourage him to breathe deeply. She encouraged him to cough and spit out any secretions, and then flush his mouth out after the treatment. Mrs. Smith wondered if the hospital was giving him a different treatment and, because it didn't seem effective, she wondered if he could have the treatments he had been getting at home. The physician checked with the nursing staff and, for the next two treatments, the drug was administered properly.*

Prevention: *The nursing staff was somewhat offended that Mrs. Smith had pointed out errors in drug administration. Because the unit was extremely understaffed, many nurses were satisfied if the patients received their medications on time, let alone had them administered following a detailed list of procedure steps. The staff didn't believe they had sufficient time to take all the steps recommended when administering a drug by nebulization.*

The patient didn't benefit from the drug when it was administered incorrectly. If it had been given correctly, he might have been discharged sooner, which would have eased the staff's workload. If a drug is going to be given, it's important to make sure that the route that's to be used is being used correctly. Prevention can be best accomplished with education and a little time.

IPPB

Intermittent positive pressure breathing (IPPB) is helpful for patients who aren't able to take deep breaths or who have restricted chest wall movement and can't breathe effectively. To administer a treatment, insert the drug into the chamber of the IPPB device and instruct the patient to sit upright, if possible. The device uses a mouthpiece or mask to deliver the drug, under pressure, to the lungs. Encourage the patient to let the machine do the work and fill the lungs. Tell him to hold his breath after each inhalation, and then to exhale normally. After treatment, encourage the patient to expectorate and to rinse his mouth to remove excess drug.

✦ Giving rectal drugs

When a patient isn't able to take drugs orally, rectal administration may be necessary. This route bypasses the digestive juices in the GI tract and the first-pass effect of biotransformation in the liver. Thus, dosage may not need to be as high as when a drug is given orally. Problems that can occur with rectal administration include poor perfusion of the area, leading to poor absorption of the drug; fecal material in the rectum, leading to poor drug absorption; or inadequate treatment if the patient can't retain the drug in the rectum long enough to allow absorption. Drugs can be administered rectally using suppositories, ointments, or enemas.

Rectal suppositories

Suppositories are bullet-shaped objects made from a substance that melts at body temperature and releases the contained drug onto the rectal mucosa for absorption. Proper administration is important for the suppository to be effective.

Instruct the patient to lie on the left side with his right knee bent. Open the suppository with a gloved hand just before insertion; don't allow the suppository to become warm and melt before insertion. Have the patient take a few deep breaths to decrease anxiety and to relax the rectal sphincter; then insert the suppository about 3″ (7.5 cm) into the rectum, so that it passes the internal sphincter. Direct it toward the side of the rectum so that it contacts the mucosal; this encourages absorption.

Urge the patient to retain the suppository for as long as possible. Many patients experience an urge to defecate when the suppository is inserted. Tell the patient to lie quietly, if possible, taking slow, deep breaths until the urge subsides. If a patient is inserting a rectal suppository himself at home, encourage him to follow the same procedure. Assess the patient's rectal area periodically to ensure that it isn't inflamed or eroded, which could alter drug absorption.

PREVENT IT

Medication error: On one medical unit, medications were prepared in one area and then passed from room to room on a medication delivery cart. A mesalamine rectal suppository was ordered for one patient, and the nurse in charge of administering medications removed one suppository from the refrigerator, and placed it on the patient's medication tray. The unit was extremely busy and the nurse had numerous interruptions. By the time she arrived at the room of the patient who needed the suppository, almost 3½ hours had passed. When the nurse removed the suppository from the foil packaging, it was very soft, and it became misshapen when she tried to insert it into the patient's rectum. Eventually, she managed to insert most of the suppository into his rectum, with a soft mass of medication remaining on the anal area and on her gloves. The patient reported being uncomfortable and, despite trying to retain the suppository, expelled the soft mass onto the bed. Both the patient and the nurse were upset with the situation, and the patient asked to see the "regular" nurse who knew how to administer the drug correctly.

Prevention: *Giving a drug rectally can be embarrassing for the patient, and every effort should be made to keep the patient calm, relaxed, and at ease. This situation could have been avoided if the nurse had used a suppository that had just been removed from the refrigerator so that it was able to melt in the rectum and not in the foil packaging. Inserting the melted mass of medication into the patient's rectum didn't deliver the drug to the rectal mucosa, but stimulated the patient's desire to defecate. If the patient is discharged with this medication, it's important to teach him that the drug should be stored in the refrigerator until just before administration.*

Rectal ointment

A rectal ointment is a semisolid medication that may be applied externally to the anus or internally to the rectum. Rectal ointments commonly contain drugs that reduce local inflammation and relieve pain and itching. When applying rectal ointment internally, be sure to lubricate the applicator to minimize discomfort on insertion. When inserting the applicator tip, direct it toward the patient's umbilicus.

Enemas

Enemas are used to flush the colon for diagnostic tests, provide drug therapy to the colon to decrease inflammation, or provide drugs to the patient for ion exchange or to stimulate rectal emptying. Some enemas come in disposable applicators with various-sized tips for adults and children, and others are delivered via an infusion container (an "enema bucket"). To decrease the cramping and peristalsis that often occurs when an enema is administered, have the patient void and empty his bowels, if possible, before administering the enema.

When giving an enema using a disposable applicator, instruct the patient to lie on the left side with his right knee bent. Ask the patient to take a deep breath as you insert the tip of the applicator into his rectum. The depth of insertion varies with the patient's age and size. Squeeze the applicator until it is empty, and encourage the patient to retain the enema for as long as indicated. When giving an enema that contains a large amount of liquid, insert the enema tubing into the rectum no more than 3", and raise the enema container until the fluid begins a steady flow into the rectum. Encourage the patient to retain the enema for as long as possible.

✦ Giving vaginal drugs

Drugs are administered into the vagina to relieve menopausal symptoms, to treat infection, to reduce inflammation, or for contraception. Vaginal preparations can take the form of suppositories, gels, foams, or creams; these come with delivery devices that make their use easier. There are several OTC preparations for treating vaginal fungal infections.

Instruct the patient to void before administering the drug. Many women prefer to insert vaginal medications themselves. If this is the preferred approach, review the procedure with your patient and suggest using a water-soluble lubricant on the applicator to ease insertion. Instruct her to assume the lithotomy position and insert the applicator, first with the tip angled down and then with the tip angled up to ensure dispersal of drug throughout the vagina. Depress the plunger to deliver the drug. Encourage the patient to remain in the lithotomy position for at least 5 to 10 minutes after insertion (30 minutes with a vaginal suppository) to allow the drug to come in contact with the vaginal walls. Check the patient's perineum periodically for abrasions and inflammation.

If the patient is at home, tell her to administer the drug at bedtime to increase retention in the vagina. Many vaginal drugs can be used during the menstrual period; however, advise the patient not to insert a tampon immediately after inserting such drugs. Recommend the use of a sanitary pad to protect the patient's underwear when such drugs are used.

PREVENT IT

Medication error: Andrea, an 18-year-old college student, was treated with antibiotics for acute cellulitis in her leg. Toward the end of her treatment, she complained of vaginal discharge, irritation, and itching. A vaginal yeast infection, most likely a superinfection related to her antibiotic therapy, was diagnosed. Andrea was prescribed clotrimazole vaginal inserts to treat the fungal infection and was asked to telephone in 3 days to report her progress. Embarrassed by her diagnosis, Andrea picked up her prescription and left the pharmacy quickly with the instruction sheet.

After 3 days, Andrea was distraught that her vaginal problem had worsened, and the nurse practitioner (NP) asked her to come in to the office for evaluation. On examination, her fungal infection did seem to be worse. While looking up other possible antifungals to try, the NP asked if Andrea had stayed in the lithotomy position for at least 30 minutes after inserting the drug. Surprised, Andrea said she had been taking the vaginal inserts orally. Because an oral drug caused the yeast infection, she thought it would be treated orally. When asked if the pharmacist or prescriber had told her how to use the drug, she responded that she hadn't heard them if they did. The NP reviewed the vaginal insertion of clotrima-zole with Andrea and asked if she had any questions about the procedure. After 3 days, Andrea reported that the symptoms were gone.

Prevention: *Many women are uncomfortable about discussing the vaginal administration of drugs. This may be more of an issue with young girls who are away at school and taking care of their own medical needs for the first time. This error could have been prevented and Andrea could have been spared extra days of suffering had she received education about the drug before she left the prescriber's office or the pharmacy. Although taking the drug orally didn't cause her any problems, she certainly didn't receive any benefit. It may seem only sensible and routine to health care providers that when a drug is ordered for vaginal administration, the patient should understand how to use it. However, routine for the provider is often unique for the patient. Patient education is essential to ensure correct drug administration.*

✦ Applying topical drugs

Drugs are administered topically to provide a local effect without their associated systemic effects. Such drugs can be used to treat inflammation, infection, or pain. Topical medications are available in several forms that affect their administration and their effect on the skin; these include lotions, creams, ointments, pastes, powders, sprays, shampoos, mouthwashes, and lozenges. Although transdermal medications are considered topical, they're discussed later in this chapter.

A key point to remember when applying a topical drug is that it's designed to act locally and not systemically. If the integrity of the area to be treated isn't intact or the area is inflamed, the drug may be absorbed systemically and possibly cause toxic effects. If the area to be treated has open or excoriated skin, withhold the drug and consult the prescriber. Also, many topical drugs shouldn't be used with occlusive dressings because these dressings can increase the risk of systemic absorption.

Before applying a topical drug, clean the treatment site and pat it dry. Apply the medication with an applicator or gloved fingers. Instruct patients who use topical medications at home to use gloves or an applicator to avoid extra exposure of the drug on their hands. Clean the site of the old drug before applying another dose.

Many OTC first-aid products are supplied as topical agents; encourage patients to read and carefully follow the directions supplied with these products. A thin layer of steroid cream on an inflamed area may relieve symptoms; however, spreading too much of the steroid cream on the area (a patient may reason that if a little makes it feel better, a lot might cure it) can cause systemic absorption and problems associated with the use of systemic steroids.

Lotion

A lotion is a solution that contains an insoluble powder suspended in water or another emulsion. When a lotion is applied, it leaves a uniform layer of powder in the film on the patient's skin. Apply medicated lotion only to affected skin areas because it may cause skin breakdown on unaffected areas.

Cream

A cream is an oil-in-water emulsion that lubricates the skin and acts as a barrier to protect the skin. It may be applied using a tongue blade to transfer the cream onto gloved fingers. Use long, smooth strokes to apply the cream evenly. As with lotion, apply medicated cream only to affected areas to prevent skin break-down of unaffected areas.

PREVENT IT

Medication error: Bonnie Rowe, age 3 months, was being evaluated for failure to thrive. The student nurse assigned to her care noted a red, oozing rash on the infant's buttocks and perineum, which was bleeding when the diaper was changed. Thinking of the pain the rash must be causing the baby, the nurse applied a liberal amount of hydrocortisone cream to the area, and then covered it with a diaper and plastic liner. Because the infant seemed less fussy, the nurse repeated the practice throughout her shift, and told the patient care assistant (PCA) assigned to the infant to continue the procedure.

This care continued for 3 days. Although the rash appeared to be improving, the infant now had complications of high blood sugar, diarrhea, muscle weakness, and rash over other parts of her body. When the tube of hydrocortisone was empty, the PCA asked the medication nurse for more. Unaware of an order for hydrocortisone cream for Bonnie, that nurse investigated. She noted that large amounts of the cream were being applied to an open, oozing area and then covered with an occlusive plastic-lined diaper, and she became concerned that the drug might have been absorbed systemically. The new problems the infant was having could have resulted from hydrocortisone absorption. The practice was stopped and the infant's diaper rash was treated with a diaper rash ointment, which repelled water and provided protection for the area while it soothed the skin.

Prevention: If the student nurse had read the instructions on the tube of hydrocortisone cream, she would have seen that it said to apply only a thin layer and to avoid occlusive dressings. She said that her mother used that type of cream and that it was "just" topical, so she didn't know that so many problems could arise from inappropriate use of the drug. The unit disposed of the extra drugs that were kept available on an as-needed basis in the unit and held a staff conference on the problems that can occur when a topical drug isn't applied correctly. Hydrocortisone cream is available over-the-counter, and it's often used by distraught parents to soothe a bad diaper rash. Caution parents to carefully read the instructions before using any drug on an infant.

Ointment

An ointment is a semisolid preparation that isn't water soluble; it helps retain heat and provides prolonged exposure of the drug to the skin. Follow the same procedure for applying an ointment as for a cream. It may be difficult to remove old ointment because of its water insolubility; be sure to use extreme care because the treatment area is already damaged. (See *Removing an ointment*.)

Never apply ointment to a patient's eyelids or ear canal unless specifically ordered because the ointment could congeal and occlude the tear duct or ear canal.

Paste

A paste is a thick preparation of powder and ointment that provides prolonged exposure of the drug to the skin and forms a protective, water-repellant barrier on the skin. Apply paste with a gloved hand in long, smooth strokes. Stroke in the direction of hair growth to avoid forcing the drug into the patient's hair follicle, which can lead to irritation and folliculitis.

Powder

A powder is an inert chemical that may contain medication; it helps keep the skin dry and reduce macera-

Removing an ointment

To remove old ointment, get a solvent, such as cottonseed oil, and some sterile 4″ × 4″ gauze pads and gloves. Wash your hands, put on the gloves, and saturate a gauze pad with some cottonseed oil, as shown below.

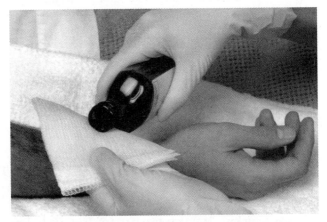

Use the saturated pad to swab the ointment gently away from the patient's skin. Rub in the direction of hair growth, and don't wipe too hard or you may irritate the skin. After you've removed the ointment, use another gauze pad to remove excess cottonseed oil. Then remove your gloves and wash your hands.

tion and friction. Make sure that the skin surface is dry before application. Shake the powder onto your gloved hand before applying a thin layer to the affected skin. Be careful that the patient doesn't inhale airborne powder, which may cause respiratory distress.

Powder aspiration can lead to severe bronchiolar obstruction after a delay of a few hours and carries a high mortality rate. A 7½-month-old infant girl developed severe respiratory distress 3 to 4 hours after aspirating powder. Intubated and maintained on a ventilator for 10 days, she suffered complications of insufficient alveolar ventilation, atelectasis, pneumonia, and superinfection. The child recovered, with some residual radiologic changes in the lungs.

Spray

A spray provides a thin film of medication to the affected area and may be delivered through an aerosol, pump, or atomizer. To spray the film evenly, hold the container 6" to 12" (15 to 30.5 cm) away from the skin. To keep the patient from inhaling aerosol, tell him to turn his head and hold his breath as the medication is being sprayed.

If using a throat spray (usually a pump), hold the nozzle just outside the patient's mouth and direct the spray to the back of the throat. Squeeze the container firmly and quickly, using enough force to propel the spray to the back of the throat.

If using an atomizer, insert the tip just inside the patient's mouth and direct the spray to the back of the throat. Advise the patient not to swallow for a few moments so that the medication can run down his throat and coat his mucous membranes. For the drug to be more effective, instruct the patient to avoid eating or drinking for at least 30 minutes after using throat spray.

Shampoo

A shampoo is a liquid solution used for its local effect on the scalp. Medicated shampoo may be used for conditions such as dandruff, psoriasis, and head lice.

Before applying the shampoo, be sure to shake the bottle well to mix the solution evenly. Apply the proper amount of shampoo as directed on the bottle. Be sure to work the shampoo into the scalp and leave on as long as directed before rinsing. Keep the shampoo away from the patient's eyes. If the shampoo accidentally gets into the eyes, irrigate them promptly with water.

Mouthwash

A mouthwash or gargle may be used to treat a condition in the patient's mouth or throat, such as stomatitis, thrush, and pharyngitis. Mouthwash should be swished in the mouth, especially over the teeth and gums. Tell the patient not to swallow it (unless specifically ordered to do so), but to spit it out. A gargle should be held at the back of the throat by tilting the head back and exhaling slowly through the solution to create a gargling effect. Again, the patient shouldn't swallow the solution. If the mouthwash or gargle contains anesthetic, warn the patient to avoid eating or drinking for 30 minutes to prevent aspiration.

Lozenge

A lozenge delivers medication to the mouth and throat as it dissolves in the mouth. Warn the patient not to chew or swallow the lozenge whole because this won't deliver the desired effect. For maximum effect, also tell the patient to avoid eating or drinking for 30 minutes after taking the lozenge.

Understanding a transdermal patch

A transdermal patch is composed of several layers. The outermost layer is
an aluminized polyester barrier that confines the drug to the patch. The next
layer is a reservoir that contains the main dose of the drug. The next layer, a
membrane, controls release of the drug from the reservoir. The innermost
adhesive layer keeps the patch on the patient's skin and holds a small
amount of drug as it moves from the patch into the skin. The dots on the illustration below show the drug slowly moving through the skin and into the
bloodstream.

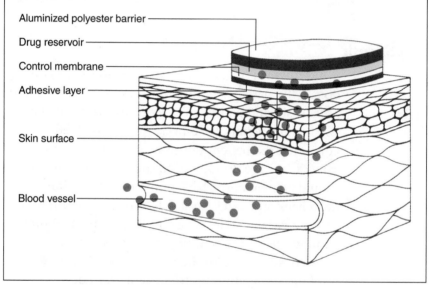

Aluminized polyester barrier

Drug reservoir

Control membrane

Adhesive layer

Skin surface

Blood vessel

◆ Applying transdermal drugs

Some drugs that were once given only orally are now
available in a slow-release system directly through the
skin.

Transdermal administration of medication achieves
a steady, prolonged, systemic effect; these drugs include hormones used for hormone replacement therapy or birth control, male hormones, nitroglycerin for
preventing angina attacks, motion sickness drugs, and

analgesic or antihypertensive medications. A transdermal drug may be supplied in a patch—which contains the drug and slowly releases it to the skin—or as an ointment applied directly to the patient's skin. (See *Understanding a transdermal patch.*) The appropriate form depends on the desired delivery time; a patch lasts longer than an ointment. Some technical aspects of using these drugs may be lost over time, so a refresher is always wise.

Transdermal patch

A transdermal patch needs to be applied to a clean, dry, hairless area of the body. Even if there's excessive hair at the chosen site, avoid shaving because it can abrade the skin and cause problems with drug absorption; however, hair may be clipped. Wash and dry the site before applying the patch. Before application, peel off the clear plastic backing without touching the adhesive side of the patch, as shown below.

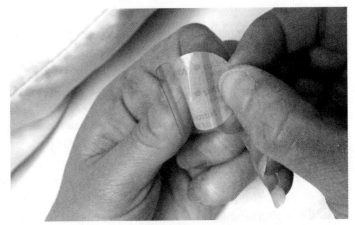

Replace the patch at regular and appropriate intervals, as indicated, to help ensure a continuous medication effect. Place the patch at a different site for each dose to avoid skin degradation and irritation. Assess the patient's skin periodically for abrasions and irritation.

Because many patients are discharged with transdermal patches, it's important to teach them how to correctly apply the drug to avoid absorption problems and loss of effectiveness. Review such teaching periodically during the course of drug therapy. Consult the manufacturer's directions for specific steps to take when a patch falls off, becomes loose, or is forgotten. The new contraceptive patch (OrthoEvra) is an example of a transdermal patch that includes a detailed list of directions for placement, replacement, and removal based on the timing of a woman's menstrual cycle.

IT'S A FACT

A critical point to remember when using a transdermal patch is that it contains an aluminized barrier. If a defibrillator is discharged onto the patch, this barrier can cause an electrical charge, resulting in arcing, smoke, and severe transdermal burns. Remove a transdermal patch in the area where a defibrillator is to be placed.

Transdermal ointment

As with a transdermal patch, apply transdermal ointment to a hairless, clean, and dry area. Because ointment is usually applied by length (for example, 2″ [5 cm] of ointment), use a measuring strip, as shown at top of next page, to ensure that the right amount of the drug is given. Patients or nurses who become comfortable with using these ointments often stop measuring the amount of ointment being used and just "eyeball" it; this practice can lead to dosing discrepancies.

Be sure to wear gloves when applying transdermal ointment to prevent drug absorption through your skin. For example, many nurses have reported headaches occurring from accidentally getting nitroglycerin cream on their skin while applying it to patients.

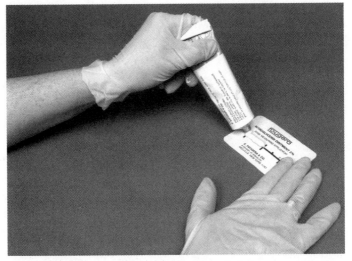

Cover the area of the application with a semipermeable dressing or a plastic wrap (also called a "patch"), as shown below, to ensure that the drug stays in contact with the skin and doesn't rub off. Tape the dressing in place, if necessary, and label the strip with the date, time, and your initials, depending on your facility's policy.

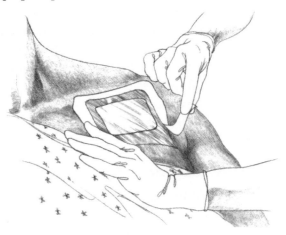

Medication error: Mr. Roskin, age 78, has a long history of coronary artery disease (CAD) and had been using nitroglycerin ointment for 2 months to prevent anginal attacks. When his wife called the clinic to inquire about the placement of the nitroglycerin ointment patch because he had "run out of room," the staff asked him to come in for an evaluation. It was discovered that Mr. Roskin had 27 nitroglycerin patches attached to different sites around his body. He didn't understand or recall being told that he was to remove the old patch before applying a new one. Some patches had been taped because they kept falling off. When removing the patches, the staff noted that the patient had developed marked irritation and reaction to the adhesive in the tape in several areas. They cared for his skin and applied a new patch to an abrasion-free area that was appropriately cleaned and dried.

Prevention: As with many medication errors, prevention can best be accomplished with proper education. Although this patient was given a printed sheet in the pharmacy when he picked up his prescription, he didn't have a direct discussion about the placement and removal of the patches. He could have had severe systemic effects from the application of so much medication. When a patient is introduced to a new delivery system for a drug, he should receive personal education as well as written material and then should demonstrate the procedure to make sure that all the important points have been understood.

✦ Giving parenteral drugs

Drugs that can't be absorbed systemically because of the nature of the drug or the patient need to be delivered directly into the body by parenteral administration. Parenteral drugs can be given intradermally (I.D.), S.C., I.M., or I.V. Such administration routes require the use of sterile techniques because they involve penetrating the body and the risk of introducing pathogens. Also, these routes aren't as convenient, cause fear in some patients, and may cause an increased risk of drug toxicity because the normal first-pass through the liver is omitted.

Intradermal injection

I.D. injection is used for administering a small amount of liquid (usually 0.5 ml or less) into the outer layer of a patient's skin. Such injections usually serve as diagnostic tests for allergies and for the standard tuberculin test.

A map should be drawn in the patient's record showing the area of the injection to facilitate reading the site for reaction after 24 to 48 hours. If you're giving more than one injection, space them about 2" (5 cm) apart. (See *Intradermal injection sites*, page 272.)

An I.D. injection uses a 26-gauge, ⅜" needle on a tuberculin syringe. (See *Giving an intradermal injection*, page 273.) Don't rub the site after the medication is injected because it may irritate the underlying tissue and alter test results. Advise the patient to avoid scratching or covering the site with a bandage. If the site gets wet, tell him to pat it dry rather than rubbing.

Subcutaneous injection

With S.C. injections, a small amount of drug (usually 0.5 to 2 ml) is injected into the S.C. tissue beneath the skin and the drug is then slowly absorbed into nearby capillaries. S.C. injections use a 25-gauge, ½" needle on an insulin or tuberculin syringe. Any area of the

Intradermal injection sites

Although the ventral forearm is usually used for I.D. injections, the upper chest, upper arm, and shoulder blades may also be used if multiple allergen tests are needed.

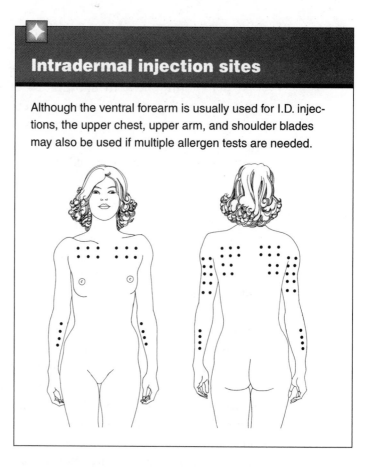

body can be used as a site for administering an S.C. injection. (See *Subcutaneous injection sites,* page 274.)

Insulin, heparin, and certain immune modulators are often given by the S.C. route. Pinch up an area of tissue, clean it with alcohol, and insert the needle at a 45-degree angle — or at a 90-degree angle for heparin and certain other drugs. When injecting heparin or insulin, avoid administration within 2″ (5 cm) of a scar, bruise, or the umbilicus. (See *Giving an S.C. injection,* page 275.)

Rotate the sites for S.C. injection to decrease the risk of abscess or necrosis. Post a rotation map in the pa-

Giving an intradermal injection

After you've selected an injection site, clean and dry the area. With one hand, stretch the skin taut; with the other hand, hold the needle at a 10- to 15-degree angle. Insert the needle just below the surface of the skin and gently inject the fluid, as shown below. Withdraw the needle at the same angle that you inserted it. A wheal or fluid-filled bump resembling a hive or blister will appear at the injection site; if it doesn't, you likely gave the injection too deep. Give another dose at least 2″ (5 cm) away from the first site.

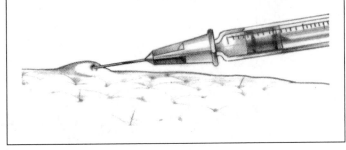

tient's record, or give it to a patient who is self-injecting at home.

S.C. administration shouldn't be used for patients in shock because the drug won't be absorbed from S.C. tissue. Monitor patients with low perfusion or blood pressure because the drug may not be absorbed or may be absorbed very slowly. For patients in a cold environment or those with chilled extremities, the resulting vasoconstriction can result in poor or absent blood flow to S.C. tissue.

PREVENT IT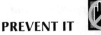

Medication error: *Mrs. Jackson, age 80, was the primary caregiver for her husband of 60 years, who had diabetes,*

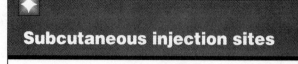

Subcutaneous injection sites

Rotate sites for subcutaneous injections to decrease the risk of formation of abscess or necrotic tissue, as shown below. The abdomen, upper thigh, and upper arm are the preferable sites for S.C. injections.

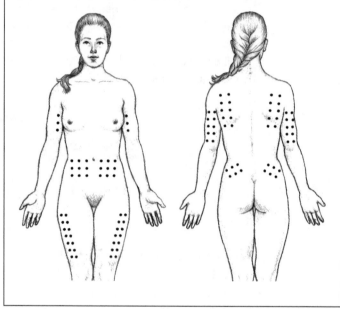

COPD, CAD, and dementia. Mrs. Jackson checked her husband's blood glucose three times a day using a fingerstick method and charted it for his physician. Over the last few weeks, she noticed that her husband's blood glucose was erratic and difficult to maintain in the desirable range. On some mornings when his blood glucose was low, she gave him glucose wafers; other days, his blood glucose was extremely high. The physician tried different insulin preparations and timings of injections without satisfying results. When the office nurse asked Mrs. Jackson if she had received training in how to check the blood and give the insulin injection, she as-

Giving an S.C. injection

To administer a subcutaneous (S.C.) injection, first select the injection site. Any area of the body that can be "pinched up" can be used as an injection site. Grasp the skin around the injection site and firmly pinch up the subcutaneous tissue to form a 1″ (2.5-cm) fat fold, as shown at right.

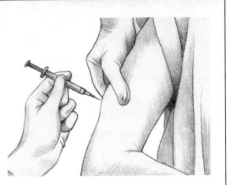

Clean the site with alcohol, then insert the needle at a 45- or 90-degree angle — as shown below — depending on the drug being administered.

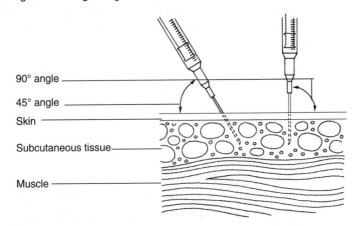

Except when administering heparin, pull back the plunger to ensure that the needle isn't in a vein; if no blood returns, inject the drug. Release the patient's skin as you inject the drug because releasing a drug into compressed tissue can irritate nerve fibers. Don't inject more than 2 ml of fluid at any one time. Massage the site gently after administering the drug, except when giving heparin or insulin.

sured her that she had. After several frustrating weeks, the physician suggested that a visiting nurse go to the patient's home to double-check the glucometer and to evaluate the living situation.

The visiting nurse arrived near lunchtime so that she could observe Mrs. Jackson check the patient's blood sugar and prepare and administer his insulin injection. Mrs. Jackson was adept at obtaining the blood sample and checking the blood glucose level. She drew up 4 units of insulin and proceeded to inject the drug directly into the deltoid muscle. When the nurse asked Mrs. Jackson about her technique in administering the drug, she learned that injection sites weren't rotated and that the same site had been used for some time. Mr. Jackson had started on insulin injections 34 years ago and the couple had then attended a five-session educational program about diabetes; they hadn't been invited to attend a refresher course since then. The visiting nurse spent much time going over how to give an S.C. injection, taking care not to upset Mrs. Jackson or make her feel that her husband's problems were caused by her technique. Over the next 2 weeks, the patient's blood glucose levels stabilized to the desired range.

Prevention: *Everyone who performs a task every day or more often over time will stop paying attention to the details of that task and it will become routine. Mrs. Jackson, based on her current attention to details, probably mastered the S.C. injection during the classes she attended with her husband. Over the years, however, her mastery had slipped and she wasn't aware that her technique was no longer correct. Student and graduate nurses are usually very aware of the proper technique for giving S.C. injections. The newness of the task and perhaps some anxiety keep the details in the forefront. Over time, however, the details may become lost—just as they did for Mrs. Jackson. There should be routine review sessions for patients, not just asking if they know how to perform a task. Staff should also periodically review techniques to pre-*

vent problems from occurring due to improper drug adminis-tration.

Intramuscular injection

An I.M. injection deposits fluid into a big muscle that has a large blood supply, which allows the drug to be absorbed quickly into the blood system. Because medication given by this route bypasses the digestive enzymes, it allows for faster action. Although up to 5 ml may be injected into a large muscle, usually 3 ml or less is given. A 20- to 23-gauge, 1" to 3" needle is used.

Sites for I.M. injections may be based on patient age and size. (See *Choosing I.M. injection sites,* pages 278 to 281.)

When giving an I.M. injection, clean the injection site with alcohol and then insert the needle quickly into the muscle. Pull back the plunger to ensure that no blood is returned, and then inject the drug. Position the patient so that his muscle is relaxed, which will aid blood flow and decrease pain.

To distract the patient and lessen pain and muscle tension, have the patient take a few deep breaths, count backwards from ten, or answer simple questions. Apply heat to the injection site to increase blood flow, aid drug absorption, and relieve pain. Some clinical centers apply ice to the injection site for immediate pain relief; this causes vasoconstriction and limits the pain-producing products in the immediate area, allowing an upset child to be driven home without tears. However, don't apply ice for an extended period of time because blood flow is needed in the area to aid drug absorption.

(Text continues on page 280.)

✦ Choosing I.M. injection sites

ADULTS

You'll usually use the deltoid, dorsogluteal, ventrogluteal, or vastus lateralis site for intramuscular (I.M.) injections.

Deltoid

Find the lower edge of the acromial process and the point on the lateral arm in line with the axilla. Insert the needle 1″ to 2″ (2.5 to 5 cm) below the acromial process, usually two or three fingerbreadths, at a 90-degree angle or angled slightly toward the process. Typical injection: 0.5 ml (range, 0.5 to 2 ml).

Ventrogluteal

Locate the greater trochanter of the femur with the heel of your hand. Spread your index and middle fingers from the anterior superior iliac spine to as far along the iliac crest as you can reach. Insert the needle between the two fingers at a 90-degree angle to the muscle. (Remove your fingers before inserting the needle.) Typical injection: 1 to 4 ml (range, 1 to 5 ml).

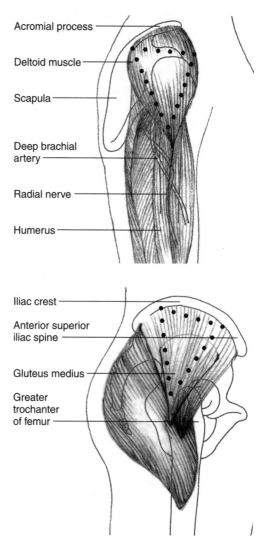

Dorsogluteal

Inject above and outside a line drawn from the posterior superior iliac spine to the greater trochanter of the femur. Alternatively, divide the buttock into quadrants and inject in the upper outer quadrant, about 2″ to 3″ (5 to 7.5 cm) below the iliac crest. Insert the needle at a 90-degree angle. Typical injection: 1 to 4 ml (range, 1 to 5 ml).

Vastus lateralis

Use the lateral muscle of the quadriceps group, from a handbreadth below the greater trochanter to a handbreadth above the knee. Insert the needle into the middle third of the muscle parallel to the surface on which the patient is lying. You may have to bunch the muscle before insertion. Typical injection: 1 to 4 ml (range, 1 to 5 ml; 1 to 3 ml for infants).

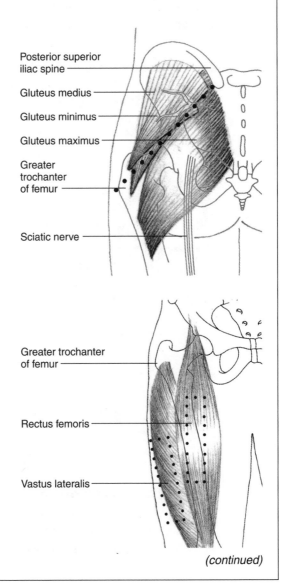

Posterior superior iliac spine

Gluteus medius

Gluteus minimus

Gluteus maximus

Greater trochanter of femur

Sciatic nerve

Greater trochanter of femur

Rectus femoris

Vastus lateralis

(continued)

Choosing I.M. injection sites *(continued)*

INFANTS AND CHILDREN

When selecting the best site for a child's I.M. injection, consider the child's age, weight, and muscular development; the amount of subcutaneous fat over the injection site; the type of drug you're administering; and the drug's absorption rate.

Vastus lateralis and rectus femoris injections

For a child under age 3, you'll typically use the vastus lateralis or rectus femoris muscle for an I.M. injection. Constituting the largest muscle mass in this age group, the vastus lateralis and rectus femoris have few major blood vessels and nerves.

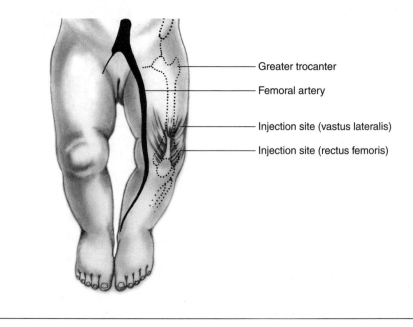

Greater trocanter

Femoral artery

Injection site (vastus lateralis)

Injection site (rectus femoris)

Z-track technique. Solutions such as iron that are very irritating to the tissues or may stain the tissues may need to be given by the Z-track technique. (See *Giving a Z-track injection*, page 282.)

Dorsogluteal and ventrogluteal injections

For a child over age 3 who has been walking for at least 1 year, you'll probably use the dorsogluteal or ventrogluteal muscle. These muscles are relatively free of major blood vessels and nerves.

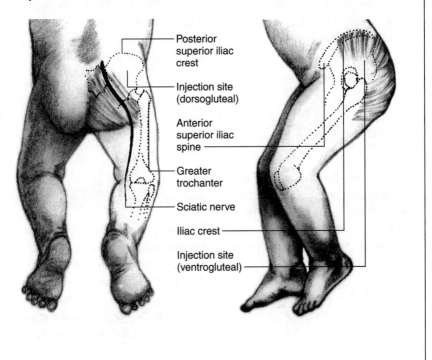

Posterior superior iliac crest

Injection site (dorsogluteal)

Anterior superior iliac spine

Greater trochanter

Sciatic nerve

Iliac crest

Injection site (ventrogluteal)

PREVENT IT

Medication error: Jason, a 28-year-old construction worker, was due for a booster tetanus shot. He told the nurse that he

✦ Giving a Z-track injection

By blocking the needle pathway after injection, the Z-track technique allows intramuscular injection while minimizing the risk of subcutaneous irritation and staining from such drugs as iron dextran. The illustrations below show how to perform a Z-track injection.

Before the procedure begins, the skin, subcutaneous fat, and muscle lie in their normal positions.

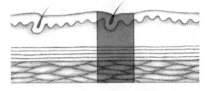

To begin, place your finger on the skin surface, and pull the skin and subcutaneous layers out of alignment with the underlying muscle. You should move the skin about ½″ (1 cm).

Insert the needle at a 90-degree angle at the site where you initially placed your finger. Inject the drug and withdraw the needle.

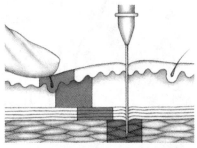

Finally, remove your finger from the skin surface, allowing the layers to return to their normal positions. The needle track (shown in the illustration by the dotted line) is now broken at the junction of each tissue layer, trapping the drug in the muscle.

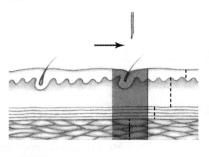

didn't want to have the shot because he remembered how painful it was in the past; he said he needed to work and couldn't cope with a sore arm. The nurse stressed the importance of getting the booster because of his work and the potential for injury and exposure to tetanus. Jason finally agreed when the nurse told him that application of an ice pack on the injection site soon after the injection appeared to dull the pain in other patients. After he received the shot in his deltoid muscle, the nurse immediately put an ice pack on the site. He commented that it didn't hurt and left for work. Three days later, Jason was seen with a hard, reddened, swollen, and painful area on his arm. It was determined that the injection site had formed an abscess and he was started on antibiotic therapy.

Prevention: *Patients should know that injections can cause pain. Jason told the staff that because the ice pack stopped the pain, he kept ice on the injection site for 2 days, applying new ice packs every few hours when they were no longer cold. The nurse hadn't thought to tell him to leave the ice on for only 20 minutes, and the patient had taken the suggestion to the extreme. The nurse felt terrible that her suggestion for relieving the patient's pain had led to an abscess and added expense and suffering. The staff at the clinic used this incident to research the use of heat versus cold after an injection. They recommended a hot pack to relieve pain because the injected solution would be absorbed more quickly and the long-term effects would be less. Also, the nurse was commended on convincing the patient to receive the injection, which could be very important to his future.*

Intravenous administration

I.V. administration is used when a drug is needed quickly, needs to reach a peak concentration rapidly, or can't be administered by any other route. Other reasons for I.V. administration include:

✦ drugs that are damaged by gastric juices
✦ drugs that are poorly absorbed by the GI tract
✦ drugs that are painful or irritating when given by another route, such as I.M. or S.C.

I.V. administration uses a 14- to 25-gauge needle. The injection site can be where any good vein is located, such as the hand, the antecubital space, or the forearm. In small children, the scalp is often used, whereas in neonates, the umbilicus vein or artery may be used. Document the site and the date of insertion. Follow facility policy regarding dressing changes and site rotation. Inspect the site frequently for possible infiltration of fluid, infection in the area such as phlebitis, and removal of the needle.

Drugs can be given I.V. by direct injection into a vein or into the injection port of I.V. tubing; or the drugs can be infused more slowly through an I.V. system into a vein by using standard I.V. solution as the vehicle to carry the drug into the vein.

Be sure to check the medication order closely. Sometimes, the abbreviations for intravenous piggyback (IVPB) and I.V. push (IVP) can be confused, and they aren't the same. IVPB refers to medication that's given over a period of time, such as an antibiotic; it can be given through a saline lock or through a secondary port on I.V. tubing. IVP refers to giving a bolus of medication through an I.V. line. Medication given in this manner produces a peak level almost immediately in the patient's blood. Misinterpreting an IVPB order and giving a drug, such as with potassium chloride, IVP can be a life-threatening error. Double-check all orders with these abbreviations.

Ensure that the drug to be injected is compatible with the I.V. solution being used or with other drugs that may be given through the same tubing. Many drugs are so sensitive that they require their own tubing and solution and can't be combined in solution, at the Y connector, or in any tubing with other drugs. A good drug guide will list the compatibilities and incompatibilities for drugs given I.V. Monitor patients closely when giving a drug I.V.; there's usually a very rapid onset of action and patients who are going to have a reaction to the drug or respond adversely to the drugs effects will usually react within a few minutes of drug administration. If the compatibility of drugs to be administered is unknown, be sure to flush the I.V. line between medications with 2 to 3 ml of saline before and after the secondary infusion.

PREVENT IT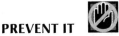

Medication error: *Andrew, 26 years old with a suspicious brain tumor, underwent a craniotomy and was moved to the ICU for close monitoring following surgery. The orders included phenytoin to prevent seizures, a common response in the early recovery period. The nurse assigned to Andrew attached a drip unit to the 5% dextrose in water that he had running, filled the chamber with 50 ml of the I.V. solution, and added the phenytoin to the chamber. She continued with his care and within a few minutes the alarm went off, indicating a problem with the infusion. She checked the site and noted that the infusion had stopped running. Following procedure, she flushed the line with saline, noted that it was again running, and restarted the medication. In a very short time, the alarm went off again. This time, the nurse carefully inspected the I.V. line and noticed that small, white crystals were forming all the way down the tubing. She immediately stopped the infusion and called her supervisor to report the problem and to decide on further action.*

Prevention: The supervisor recognized that the problem was with the phenytoin and the I.V. solutions. Referring to her drug guide, the supervisor showed the nurse that phenytoin shouldn't be mixed with dextrose solutions. For I.V. use, the drug should be given by slow I.V. push of not more than 40 mg/minute. The dextrose and the phenytoin interacted to

*cause crystallization. Luckily, the patient didn't suffer any
seizures and a new I.V. line was established. The nurse posted
a notice on the patient's chart and above his bed reminding
other staff about phenytoin's incompatibility with dextrose solutions and its need to be given by I.V. push. The supervisor
used this incident to organize a staff education meeting that
reviewed the drugs they commonly used that shouldn't be
mixed with certain I.V. solutions or other drugs. It's important to have refresher sessions on drug compatibility issues, especially when staff and the drugs being used change so frequently.*

Giving an intermittent infusion

An intermittent drug infusion is given for a short time
through a secondary administration set or a volume-
controlled set. Some primary administration sets have
several ports through which these infusions are connected. Before connecting an intermittent infusion,
know the difference with using these ports.

To infuse a piggyback drug without also infusing the
primary infusion, hang the piggyback container above
the level of the primary I.V. solution, using the extension set that's supplied with the piggyback infusion set.
Then connect the extension to the port closest to the
top of the administration set (closest to the primary I.V.
infusion). Using a lower port on the primary administration set won't stop the infusion of the primary I.V.
By infusing the primary and secondary solutions si-
multaneously, you may cause fluid overload. For example, a heart failure patient with a keep-vein-open
rate of I.V. fluids is prescribed Bactrim, which is mixed
in 250 ml of fluid, to be given over 2 hours. This increase in fluid may cause fluid overload. Or, if the patient is volume depleted and needs I.V. fluids, you may
be drastically decreasing the prescribed fluid administration for the amount of time that an I.V. medication

is ordered. For example, a patient who had a GI hemorrhage and is receiving I.V. fluids at 250 ml per hour, suddenly drops to 50 ml an hour during the administration of an antibiotic. These outcomes must be considered when giving I.V. intermittent infusions. If the primary infusion can't be interrupted to run an incompatible secondary infusion, consider a double-lumen catheter or starting another I.V. line. (See *Using a piggyback set*, page 288.)

Infiltrated medications. Because of patient movement and factors such as multiple types of equipment in use and the condition of the patient's veins, the integrity of an I.V. line may be compromised. Be sure to monitor all I.V. sites, especially when administering drugs that may be toxic to tissues, such as dopamine or calcium. If a medication infiltrates, be sure to contact the pharmacy regarding antidotes that may be recommended to decrease tissue damage. Also, when a medication begins infusing into the tissue, the patient may not be receiving the full effect of the drug, and may begin displaying a response to this situation.

PREVENT IT

Medication error: Dave Jones, a 48-year-old male admitted to the ER after experiencing crushing chest pain, was diagnosed with an acute inferior wall myocardial infarction. He was started on a nitroglycerin drip, which resolved his chest pain. After transfer to the cardiac intensive care, he began to complain again of chest pain. Although the nurse increased his nitroglycerin drip as ordered, his pain increased. The cardiac monitor began showing changes in his heart rhythm and he became diaphoretic and short of breath. The nurse continued to increase the nitroglycerin drip as she obtained an electrocardiogram. Finally, the nurse was ordered to give morphine sulfate I.V. When she went to administer the drug, she noticed

Using a piggyback set

A piggyback set is useful for intermittent drug infusion. So as not to infuse I.V. fluids while administering medication, the secondary set's container must be positioned higher than the primary set's container.

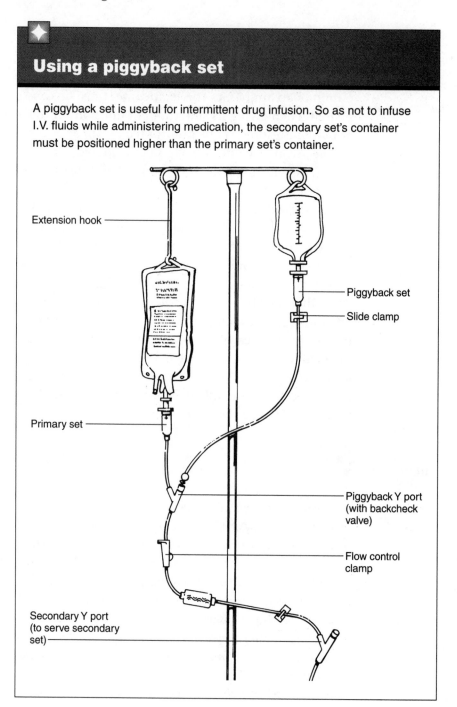

Extension hook

Primary set

Secondary Y port (to serve secondary set)

Piggyback set

Slide clamp

Piggyback Y port (with backcheck valve)

Flow control clamp

that his I.V. was severely infiltrated. She quickly started another I.V., administered the morphine, and restarted the nitroglycerin drip. Mr. Jones' chest pain subsided and his heart rhythm returned to normal.

* **Prevention:** This situation could have been resolved quickly if the nurse had checked the I.V. site when she increased the nitroglycerin drip. Much movement, such as when the patient is transferred from the ER stretcher to the bed in the cardiac unit, may cause dislodgment of the I.V. catheter. Careful monitoring of the site can prevent medication or fluid from infiltrating into the tissue.*

Intraosseous administration

Intraosseous administration is the delivery of medication, fluid, or blood into the bone marrow. It's used for emergency situations, usually involving infants or children. To administer a drug by this route, insert an intraosseous needle into the anterior surface of the bone, usually the tibia. Any drug that can be given I.V. can be given by intraosseous infusion with comparable absorption and effectiveness. Be sure to check for extravasation of fluid into S.C. tissue. Discontinue intraosseous infusion as soon as conventional vascular access is established. (See *Understanding intraosseous infusion*, page 290.)

Knowing all the tubes

Patients may have a number of tubes and lines at a given time — including chest tubes, endotracheal tubes, NG tubes, feeding tubes, central lines, I.V. lines, epidural catheters, bladder catheters, and suprapubic catheters. When a drug is ordered to be given via one of these tubes, it's important to make sure that the

Understanding intraosseous infusion

During intraosseous infusion, the bone marrow serves as a noncollapsible vein; thus, fluid infused into the marrow cavity rapidly enters the circulation by way of an extensive network of venous sinusoids. The illustration below shows the needle positioned in the patient's tibia.

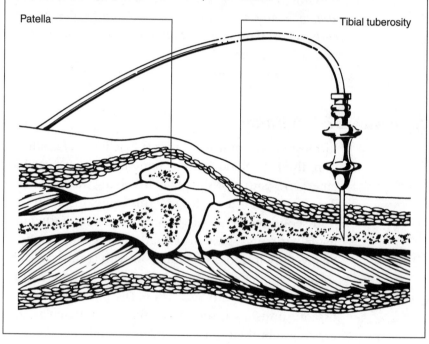

Patella — — Tibial tuberosity

tube has been correctly identified before injecting the drug. There have been reports of I.V. drugs being inadvertently delivered into tracheostomy cuff ports, causing airway occlusion; patients receiving epidural drugs have inadvertently had bladder irrigant infused into the epidural space; and patients with constant feeding through a NG tube have had their tubes clamped during administration of oral medications and then neglected.

PREVENT IT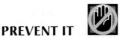

Medication error: Thirty-eight-year-old Thomas Saunders was admitted to the ICU postoperatively for multiple traumatic injuries sustained in a motorcycle accident. His injuries included multiple facial fractures, a fractured left femur, and a left hemothorax. Mr. Saunders was intubated with a #8 Shiley low-pressure tracheostomy tube due to his multiple facial fractures and obstruction of his upper airway. He also had a triple-lumen I.V. catheter inserted via the right subclavian route, and a #28 chest tube inserted into the right chest wall and connected to 20 cm H_2O wall suction. Due to a bed shortage, Mr. Saunders was transferred to a general surgical floor with his tubes in place. His new nurse was given a quick verbal report upon transfer, and a patient care assistant quickly settled Mr. Saunders in. She left the lights low, kept her patient assessment brief, and hung his regular dose of I.V. antibiotic.

Mr. Saunders appeared to be doing well and denied any difficulties. Within 30 minutes, however, he became restless and went into respiratory arrest and the code team was called. Initially, they were unable to inflate his lungs and discovered that the antibiotic had inadvertently been connected to the pilot of the Shiley low-pressure tracheostomy tube, causing the cuff to become greatly overinflated and obstruct the airway. The antibiotic was stopped, and the fluid was removed from the tracheostomy cuff.

Prevention: The key to preventing this type of error is staff orientation and education. Often, as hospitals are forced to make cuts under cost constraints, they look to staffing levels as well as nurse education and orientation as areas for significant cost savings. Moreover, nurses are often required to float to unfamiliar units to offset deficits in staffing levels. Make sure you're completely familiar with any devices that you may have to deal with. Complete a thorough assessment on *every patient. Clearly identify all devices and access lines, properly label and secure each access line, and check a line's identity each time you access it. When hanging an I.V. total parenteral nutrition or medication, always follow the tube you are using back to the source — is it going into a vein, a central port, or another piece of equipment? Make sure you're delivering the solution to the correct place. A few minutes of extra effort can save a lot of time and problems later.*

Be assertive to protect your patients. Insist that proper education and orientation be provided for any device that may be unfamiliar to you. If you're working in an unfamiliar unit, make sure you become familiar with the acuity of the patients in the unit, as well as any devices they may have.

The key point to remember when approaching a patient with any lines or tubes is to always check it out — follow the tube or line to the point of insertion, and make sure the lights are on so that all portals and tubes can be seen clearly. If a tube or line leads to an unfamiliar device, ask for guidance on how to use it to avoid problems.

✦ Replay: The fourth right

The fourth right in the commonsense approach to preventing medication errors is to make sure that the right route is used. This means first ensuring that the route that has been ordered is the route that's being used; that the route is appropriate for this patient; that the prescribed drug is available in the form that has been ordered; and that proper administration technique is used. If it has been a while since you administered a drug via an NG tube or intradermally or ophthalmically, review the technique. Details of certain techniques may be lost if not used frequently. Never

Checklist for the right route

Use the checklist below to prevent medication errors related to administration route.

PRESCRIBER'S ORDER
- ☐ Was the handwriting interpreted correctly?
- ☐ Was the verbal order understood correctly?
- ☐ Were confusing abbreviations used?

AVAILABLE FORMS
- ☐ Is the drug available in a form that can be given by the route ordered?
- ☐ If the drug needs to be altered (cut, crushed, or chewed) to be given by the route indicated, can that be done safely?

APPROPRIATENESS FOR THIS PATIENT
- ☐ Can the patient safely take the drug by the ordered route?
- ☐ Can the patient swallow oral medications?
- ☐ Does the patient have good peripheral perfusion for an S.C. or I.M. injection?
- ☐ Is the patient cold, which could interfere with absorption of injected drugs?
- ☐ Does the patient have erosions or lesions at the site intended for topical, buccal, sublingual, nasal, vaginal, or rectal administration?

TECHNIQUE
- ☐ Have you reviewed the correct technique for administering the drug by this route?

assume that administration is easy and anyone can do it: When in doubt, check it out. (See *Checklist for the right route*.)

Chapter

7

The right time

The fifth "right" to consider before administering a drug is whether you're giving the drug at the right time. This means assuring that the timing ordered for doses of the drug has been interpreted correctly, that the time the drug is to be given doesn't conflict with the presence of another drug or food that could interfere with the drug's effects, and that the drug is actually delivered within the time frame that will provide its greatest therapeutic effect. This last aspect is challenging in a busy health care facility where distractions for the nursing staff include scheduled tests and procedures for patients and a myriad of scheduled therapies and tasks that can interfere with drug delivery.

✦ Therapeutic timing

Timing of drug administration can play a critical role in determining whether a drug dose will be therapeutic, ineffective, or toxic. A review of the pharmacokinetics of drugs in the body helps to explain the importance of proper timing.

Critical concentration

After a drug is administered, its molecules must first be absorbed into the body and then make their way to the reactive tissues. If a drug is going to work properly on these reactive tissues—thus having a therapeutic effect—it has to reach a high enough concentration in the body. The amount of a drug needed to cause a therapeutic effect is called the *critical concentration.*

Drug evaluation studies determine the critical concentration required to cause the desired therapeutic effect. The recommended dosage of a drug is based on the amount that needs to be given to eventually reach the critical concentration. Excessive concentration produces toxic effects, whereas too little doesn't produce the desired therapeutic effects.

The actual concentration that a drug reaches in the body results from a dynamic equilibrium that involves several factors:

✦ absorption from the site of entry
✦ distribution to the active site
✦ biotransformation (metabolism) in the liver
✦ excretion from the body.

These factors are key elements in determining the amount of drug needed (dose) and the frequency of the dose repetition (scheduling) required to reach the critical concentration for the desired length of time. When administering a drug, consider the phases of pharmacokinetics to try to make the drug regimen as effective as possible. Has the patient just eaten? This would affect absorption. Is the room too cold? This could affect blood flow and distribution. Does the patient have adequate liver function that isn't being influenced by other drugs or foods? This could affect metabolism. Does the patient have adequate renal function that isn't being influenced by other drugs, foods, or blood flow problems that will encourage drug excretion? These factors need to be balanced to provide the patient the best chance of getting the therapeutic effects of the drug with the least chance of adverse effect. (See *Drug distribution,* page 296.)

Drug distribution

Drug disposition begins as soon as a drug is administered. The drug proceeds through pharmacokinetic, pharmacodynamic, and pharmacotherapeutic phases. The chart below shows the phases, the activities that occur during them, and the factors that influence those actions.

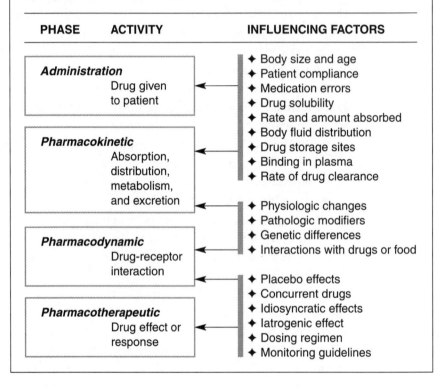

PHASE	ACTIVITY	INFLUENCING FACTORS
Administration	Drug given to patient	✦ Body size and age ✦ Patient compliance ✦ Medication errors ✦ Drug solubility ✦ Rate and amount absorbed
Pharmacokinetic	Absorption, distribution, metabolism, and excretion	✦ Body fluid distribution ✦ Drug storage sites ✦ Binding in plasma ✦ Rate of drug clearance
Pharmacodynamic	Drug-receptor interaction	✦ Physiologic changes ✦ Pathologic modifiers ✦ Genetic differences ✦ Interactions with drugs or food
Pharmacotherapeutic	Drug effect or response	✦ Placebo effects ✦ Concurrent drugs ✦ Idiosyncratic effects ✦ Iatrogenic effect ✦ Dosing regimen ✦ Monitoring guidelines

Half-life

A drug's half-life is the time it takes for the amount of drug in the body to decrease to one-half of the peak level it previously achieved. For example, if a patient takes 20 mg of a drug with a half-life of 2 hours, 10 mg of the drug will remain 2 hours after administration. Two hours later, 5 mg will be left (one-half of

What's half-life?

Your patient's drug dosage depends on its half-life—the time it takes for the drug's level in the blood to fall to half its peak. The diagram below shows the time required (2½ hours) for the blood level of gentamicin, given by I.V. injection, to fall to 3 mcg/ml—half its peak level of 6 mcg/ml. Blood samples taken at specific intervals reveal how much of the drug remains in the patient's bloodstream. This information helps to establish how much of a drug to give, and how often, to maintain a therapeutic blood level.

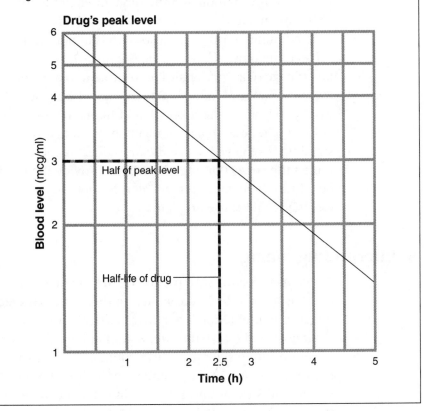

Drug's peak level

Half of peak level

Half-life of drug

Blood level (mcg/ml)

Time (h)

the previous level); and in 2 more hours, only 2.5 mg will remain. This is important to determine the appropriate timing for a drug dose or the timing of a drug's effect on the body. (See *What's half-life?*)

A drug's half-life is determined by a balance of all the factors at work on that drug: absorption, distribution, biotransformation, and excretion. The absorption rate, speed of biotransformation, distribution to the tissues, and rate of drug excretion are taken into consideration when determining the half-life of a drug. The half-life given in a drug monograph is that for a healthy person. The prescriber can use this information to estimate the half-life of a drug for a patient with kidney or liver dysfunction (which could prolong the biotransformation and the time for excretion of a drug) and make changes in the dosage schedule.

The timing of drug administration is important to achieve the most effective drug therapy. Use your knowledge of a drug's half-life to explain to a patient the importance of following a schedule of drug administration either in the hospital or at home. It's easier to enforce schedules in a drug regimen when this understanding is achieved. Once the prescriber has determined the correct timing of a drug to provide the most benefit to the patient, remain alert for potential obstacles that could cause problems.

✦ Interpreting timing

Problems involving interpreting the timing of a drug that has been ordered are similar to those encountered when trying to decide what drug has been ordered at what dose and by what route. Poor handwriting, poor communication skills, and distractions can lead to a misinterpretation of the intended timing that has been ordered. Misuse or misunderstanding of abbreviations is a major problem that occurs with timing orders. (See *Abbreviations that cause timing errors.*)

Abbreviations that cause timing errors

Certain abbreviations that involve timing have been reported to result in medication errors. Here are some common examples, with tips for prescribers:

✦ *once daily* — abbreviated as q.d., QD, OD, or o.d. The usual accepted abbreviation is q.d.; however, this has frequently been misread as "qid" (four times a day), which could result in a serious overdose. O.D. (once daily) has been misinterpreted to mean "right eye." Reports also cite the misunderstanding of qd (each day) as "each dose," which could lead to serious overdose. *Tip:* Write out "daily" or "every day" to avoid such errors.

✦ *every other day* — abbreviated q.o.d. or QOD. This has reportedly been misinterpreted to mean qd (daily) or qid (four times a day). Some abbreviation lists don't even recognize qod. *Tip:* Write out "every other day" when this dosage is needed.

✦ *nightly at bedtime* — often abbreviated qhs (at the hour of sleep), which has been misread as "every hour." This phrase is sometimes written as "qn" for every night, often misinterpreted as "qh" (every hour). Some reports cite "BT" being used as an abbreviation for "bedtime," misinterpreted to mean "bid" (twice daily). *Tip:* Write out "nightly" or "at bedtime" if that's the intended timing of the drug dose.

✦ *every day at a specific time* — for example, q4 p.m. — has been misinterpreted to mean every 4 hours. *Tip:* If a drug is ordered to be given every day at a specific time, write it out to avoid confusion — every day at 4 p.m. — instead of combining convenient abbreviations to get the message across.

✦ *at discharge* — often abbreviated D/C, which is also used to mean "discontinue." Many errors have occurred when a patient is to be given medications or medication orders at discharge and they are inadvertently discontinued. It's important to clarify what's meant by D/C any time the abbreviation is used. When in doubt, check it out.

Medication error: A patient with valvular heart disease was discharged to home with the following prescription: clopidogrel (Plavix) 75 mg PO q.d. The secretary who transcribed the order to the discharge papers read the prescription as 75 mg PO qid, or four times a day. The nurse who reviewed the discharge paperwork was extremely busy and anxious to get the patient discharged to make room for another, and reported later that she wasn't familiar with Plavix. The pharmacist who received the prescription became concerned that the dose was much higher than he had seen previously. He checked with the prescriber who insisted that he had written "qd," meaning "each day," and not "qid." The prescription was corrected and the order filled. The next day, the prescriber went to the unit to determine what had happened. When he looked at his handwriting, he saw that the period after "q" resembled a small "i."

Prevention: Luckily, the patient suffered no ill effects from the drug order. Although it's easy to see how the error was made, in retrospect, it would be difficult to teach all health care providers how to prevent this type of abbreviation error. The staff at this unit decided that "once a day," "each day," or "per day" should be written out on all prescriptions. Prescribers who felt it would be time-consuming asked that they be allowed to write the prescription with "dose/d"—such as 75 mg/d PO—because this would also avoid confusion. Working together, the nurses and prescribers were able to devise a method that would avoid repetition of the medication error.

✦ Interactive timing

Some drugs are known for interacting with each other and causing potential problems for the patient. These drugs often have to be spaced during the day so that they aren't in the stomach at the same time. For example, tetracycline absorption is blocked by the presence of iron, zinc, antacids, calcium, and urinary alkalinizers. If tetracycline is to be given to a patient taking any of these drugs, stagger it around the other drugs to prevent problems. Because antacids can change the pH of the gastric contents and alter the breakdown and absorption of several drugs, always schedule it away from other drugs. (See *Drug interactions*, page 302.)

The effect of food

Certain drugs are affected by the presence of food in the stomach. Food stimulates the release of gastric acid and causes a slowing of gastric emptying. This can hasten the premature breakdown of drugs in the stomach because of the increased acid and the drug's prolonged exposure to it. Drugs that are sensitive to such effects often come with a caution to take the drug on an empty stomach — 1 hour before or 2 hours after meals — and usually with water. If your patient is going home with such a drug, give him written instructions for taking it.

Some drugs are better absorbed if food is present in the stomach; such drugs are usually specified to be taken with food. Unless you work daily with these drugs, the only way to know which ones should or shouldn't be taken with food is to refer to a timely drug guide. Drug administration can be challenging if a patient is taking several drugs — some that have to be taken alone, on an empty stomach, and others that have to be taken with food. Keeping the drugs organized and administered at the correct time is the only way to ensure that the patient receives the drug's best therapeutic effect with the least toxic reaction.

Drug interactions

Some drugs are known for interacting with each other and causing potential problems for the patient. The chart below lists types of drug interactions.

INTERACTION	CHARACTERISTICS
Indifference	✦ This is the most common type of drug interaction. ✦ Both drugs promote the action of the most active component of the combination. ✦ Interaction doesn't alter the therapeutic effect of either drug or produce unpredictable adverse effects.
Additive interaction	✦ Total effect of the two drugs together equals the sum of the drug's separate effects. ✦ Some additive interactions are intended and desirable; for example, aspirin and codeine may be prescribed together to enhance pain relief. ✦ Unplanned additive interactions can have adverse effects, causing extreme sedation or other dangerous conditions.
Synergistic interaction	✦ One drug increases the other's effects, causing a total effect greater than the sum of the drug's separate effects. ✦ Like an additive interaction, synergism may be beneficial or harmful.
Antagonistic interaction	✦ One drug interferes with the other's actions, negating its therapeutic value. ✦ An example is levodopa and pyridoxine (vitamin B_6) administered simultaneously. Normally, levodopa reduces stiffness, rigidity, and other symptoms of Parkinson's disease, but because pyridoxine antagonizes it, the patient may not receive levodopa's therapeutic actions.

PREVENT IT

Medication error: Mrs. Avery, age 86, moved into a skilled nursing facility when she became unable to care for herself safely in her own home. She had rheumatic fever as a child and subsequent mitral valve disease. She has had heart failure for several years and has been stable on her regimen of digoxin (Lanoxin) 0.25 mg/day PO and furosemide (Lasix) 40 mg PO every other day for almost 12 years. Before being admitted to the facility, she was seen by her primary care provider; her laboratory tests were good and her digoxin level was within normal limits at 1.1 ng/ml.

Three weeks after entering the facility, Mrs. Avery began to develop progressive weakness, dyspnea on exertion, two-pillow orthopnea, and 2+ pitting edema peripherally. Her heart failure became progressively worse. Five days after her symptoms worsened, she was in acute heart failure and was transferred to the hospital. On admission, her physical examination revealed the signs of heart failure; her serum digoxin level was 0.12 ng/ml (therapeutic range, 0.5 to 2 ng/ml). Mrs. Avery was diuresed and her digoxin levels were restabilized.

Although she recovered well, the staff was concerned about returning her to the nursing home without knowing the cause of her problems. The patient confirmed that she was getting the same digoxin pill every day that she had taken at home. A check of the nursing home's medication records for Mrs. Avery revealed that she had received the right drug at the right dose and at the same time each day. While thinking of other factors that might have changed, the patient recalled that, at home, she had taken her digoxin each morning with a glass of water; at the nursing home she was given the drug in the afternoon. She also noted that the nursing home staff always ground up the digoxin and put it in a cup of ice *cream. Mrs. Avery thought this practice strange because she didn't have any trouble swallowing pills.*

Consultation with the clinical pharmacologist answered the riddle of Mrs. Avery's declining digoxin levels. Being cold, ice cream causes a vasoconstriction in the stomach and a slowing of muscle contractions; it also stimulates gastric acid secretion in the stomach. The combination of these two factors — increased acid and increased time in the stomach — led to a breakdown of the digoxin before it could be absorbed. The patient's digoxin levels fell over a steady period of time until they were so low that the patient no longer received the therapeutic effect needed to control her heart failure symptoms.

***Prevention:** Digoxin has a small margin of safety, or the range in which it is therapeutic versus toxic or ineffective. In Mrs. Avery's case, the change in the drug's timing and administration led to a change in its absorption by the body. The mixture of the drug with the ice cream — a routine practice at the nursing home to ensure that residents got calcium each day — caused the patient's problems. However, convincing the skilled nursing facility that this was the cause of the patient's problem was difficult.*

The old refrain, "We've always done it this way," makes introducing new thoughts or practices difficult, especially if they come from an "outsider." Mrs. Avery didn't want to upset the nurses, and the hospital staff didn't want Mrs. Avery to undergo this experience again. The hospital staff coordinated an educational program with the skilled nursing facility staff on the premise that the hospital staff had learned new clinical information and was excited to share it with them. Awareness and education can prevent this type of error from repeating itself.

The grapefruit juice dilemma

Another issue that has gained much attention is the interaction of grapefruit juice with a number of drugs. Grapefruit juice inhibits the cytochrome CYP-3A4 sys-

Grapefruit juice interactions

The chart shown below lists some drugs that shouldn't be given with grapefruit juice.

TYPE OF DRUG	SPECIFIC DRUG
Benzodiazepines	alprazolam, midazolam, triazolam
Calcium channel blockers	diltiazem, felodipine, nimodipine, nifedipine, nisoldipine, verapamil
Chemotherapeutic agents	cyclophosphamide, ifosfamide, tamoxifen, vincristine, vinblastine
HMG-CoA reductase inhibitors	atorvastatin, fluvastatin, lovastatin, pravastatin, simvastatin
HIV protease inhibitors	amprenavir, indinavir, nelfinavir, ritonavir, saquinavir
Immunosuppressives	cyclosporine A, tacrolimus
Macrolide antibiotics	clarithromycin, erythromycin, troleandomycin
Opioids	alfentanil, fentanyl, sufentanil
Steroids	budesonide, cortisol, 17 beta-estradiol, progesterone, testosterone
Other drugs	quinidine, sildenafil

tem in the liver, which can cause a decrease in the metabolism of many drugs. Decreasing the metabolism of the drug can lead to increased serum drug levels and toxicity. (See *Grapefruit juice interactions.*)

IT'S A FACT

Studies have shown that terfenadine or astemizole and grape-fruit juice may cause problems with heart rhythm. Terfena-dine-containing products were withdrawn from the market in the United States by the Food and Drug Administration in February 1998. Astemizole was withdrawn from the market in the United States and Canada by the manufacturer in June 1999.

Many people drink grapefruit juice every day. It's thought to decrease the risk of contracting the common cold and flu, decrease cholesterol levels, help in weight loss, and prevent cancer. Grapefruit juice isn't regarded as a drug or an herb, but a common breakfast drink. Because it can affect the levels of many drugs and potentially lead to toxic effects, advise patients to avoid drinking grapefruit juice if they are taking such drugs. If a patient develops toxic levels of one of these drugs, ask him about his consumption of grapefruit juice. In facilities that allow patients to select their own menus, caution patients receiving these drugs not to select grapefruit juice as their beverage.

PREVENT IT

Medication error: *Christopher Smith's hypertension was controlled with diet, exercise, and nifedipine (Procardia). In early winter, he called his physician complaining of dizziness, light-headedness, and confusion. He was asked to come in for an examination, which revealed a pulse of 112 beats/minute and blood pressure of 94/60 mm Hg; his controlled blood pressure was normally 130/82 mm Hg. The patient denied having diarrhea or vomiting, and his skin didn't show signs*

of dehydration. His electrocardiogram revealed sinus tachy-
cardia. The patient denied the use of other drugs or herbs; the
only change in his usual routine was that he had started
drinking a few glasses of grapefruit juice each morning to
ward off colds and flu. The staff researched nifedipine in a
drug guide and found that its metabolism is inhibited by
grapefruit juice. By taking the drug with grapefruit juice in
the morning, the patient had inhibited its metabolism; the in-
creased serum levels of the drug caused the hypotension and
presenting symptoms.

*   **Prevention:** Mr. Smith was upset that he hadn't been*
warned not to drink grapefruit juice when taking this drug.
In checking with the pharmacy that filled his prescription, the
staff found that the printout given to him did mention the
avoidance of grapefruit juice, but the patient stated that he
threw away the printouts because they were confusing. He as-
sumed that if there were an important warning associated
with the drug, someone would have told him directly. The
staff in the physician's office used this experience to develop a
teaching poster for the waiting room and to have an in-service
program because the office staff admitted that they didn't
know about the grapefruit juice issue.

✦ Getting the timing right

The reality of clinical practice is that schedules have to
be established that best fit the routine of the facility.
For example, with 28 patients taking a total of 115
drugs each day and only one medication nurse to administer them, thinking that each patient will have an
individualized schedule based on his preferences and
needs is unrealistic. Most facilities have standardized
schedules — medications given at 10 a.m., 2 p.m., 6
p.m., and 10 p.m. If a patient's medications and guidelines for administration are reviewed, this may more
closely resemble a medication schedule for 9 a.m., 11

a.m., 1 p.m., 3 p.m., 4 p.m., 7 p.m., and before bed-time. Unfortunately, nurses often have to settle for do-ing the best they can under the circumstances of short staffing, sick patients, and shift changes.

During discharge, it's important to sit down with the patient and plan a medication schedule that doesn't in-terfere with his lifestyle, but follows the guidelines for timing his drug administration. Discharge is usually a busy and overwhelming time for both the patient and staff, and the patient is often given several prescrip-tions and discharged. Many patients report receiving no drug education when discharged from a facility and, if they have several pills to take each day, it's easi-est for them to take them all at once. This practice can lead to serious problems in the overall medical regi-men of the patient. If a patient is supposed to be taking an antibiotic twice a day to achieve an average critical concentration during the day but takes both doses to-gether in the morning, he will have a period of a high, potentially toxic, concentration of the drug and then a much lower-than-needed drug level later in the day, which in turn will allow bacteria to grow and continue to cause disease.

Many drug companies are working on sustained-release products that allow for once-a-day dosing. Meanwhile, if your patient is taking a drug that re-quires doses spaced throughout the day, give him spe-cific information about the timing. Filling a pillbox with the timing labeled, marking a calendar with times, or developing a medication clock as a teaching tool can also serve as useful reminders. Some patients use alarm clocks to alert them when to take a drug.

Common pitfalls

Sometimes your best efforts to maintain the right tim-ing are thwarted by events beyond your control.

The inconvenient dose

It isn't uncommon for a medication nurse to arrive at a patient's room to find that he's out of the room for therapy or a diagnostic test. Often, when the drug is to be given orally, the nurse may leave the cup containing the drug at the bedside table for the patient to take when he returns. When the patient is on the telephone or in the bathroom, the nurse may sometimes leave the medication for him to take when it's convenient. *However, this should never happen.* Leaving the medication and then charting that you administered it is considered a serious incident.

PREVENT IT

Medication error: The evening medication nurse brought a chloral hydrate capsule to Mr. Brown. He had an order for 500 mg PO at bedtime each night to help him sleep. The patient was talking on the telephone and motioned the nurse to leave the medication on his bedside table. She obliged, not wanting to interrupt his phone call. Two days later, the patient care assistant was making Mr. Brown's bed while he was undergoing tests and found six choral hydrate capsules in his pillowcase. When the charge nurse checked his medication record, she noted that his medication had been signed for each night of his stay; however, she was curious where he had obtained the drugs. The situation was discussed with the patient when he returned from his test. Eventually, Mr. Brown confessed that each evening he would have the nurse leave the capsule for him to take later and then he would hide the capsule. He admitted that he was stockpiling the capsules for a suicide attempt.

Prevention: This error wouldn't have happened if the medication nurse had stayed with Mr. Brown and observed him taking the medication. In addition, by signing the med-

*ication record, the medication nurse had created a legal state-
ment that the patient had actually received the drug. The
charge nurse used this experience as a training tool rather
than a punishment. All the unit's nurses participated in an
in-service program on safe medication practices.*

*Never leave drugs at a patient's bedside unless he has spe-
cific orders for it to be left there. A nurse administering a drug
needs to make sure that the drug has been successfully given
before she signs the legal record for that patient. When units
are busy and understaffed, these errors may occur. Taking the
time to ensure that a drug has been administered correctly
and at the right time, however, can save many hours of paperwork and future patient problems.*

Combining drugs

In health care facilities, it's sometimes necessary to
combine drugs to ensure that the patient gets all the
medications that have been ordered for him for the
day. As discussed in chapter 6, the combination of
drugs can lead to problems that may prolong the illness or cause additional adverse effects for the patient.

PREVENT IT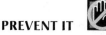

*Medication error: Mary King, age 52, was admitted
through the emergency department with a compound fracture
of the left leg, the result of a skiing accident. Her left femur
and tibia were fractured in several places. The leg was set sur-
gically and she was admitted to the orthopedic unit with full
leg traction. An order was written to resume her regular medications, which included levothyroxine (Synthroid) 0.125 mg
daily for hypothyroidism and alendronate (Fosamax) 10 mg/
day for preventing postmenopausal osteoporosis. When the
nurse came to administer these medications the morning after
surgery, Ms. King told her that she couldn't take the Fosamax*

unless she could sit upright for 30 minutes and that she couldn't take both the pills together because the Fosamax had to be taken on an empty stomach. Ms. King wasn't able to sit upright because of the angle of the traction. The overworked nurse assured the patient that everything would be fine and that the patient had to take both drugs together or else the nurse might not be able to give them to her until late afternoon.

By the third day, the patient complained of severe epigastric pain and was having difficulty swallowing. Diagnostic studies revealed that she had several small erosions in her esophagus that had developed during her hospital stay. She was started on cimetidine (Tagamet) 1600 mg daily and the Fosamax was discontinued. Ms. King reported that since she had been hospitalized, she hadn't followed her routine of taking the Fosamax on an empty stomach with a full glass of water and staying upright for 30 minutes. The pharmacist had given her these strict instructions when she first received her prescriptions and she followed them closely. Because the hospital nurse had reassured her, the patient thought that the pharmacist might have been overemphasizing a precaution that might be unnecessary in a hospital situation where constant care is given.

Prevention: *Alendronate (Fosamax) belongs to a class of drugs called bisphosphonates that work to promote calcium deposition in bone and are used for the prevention and treatment of postmenopausal osteoporosis and for treating Paget's disease. These drugs can be extremely erosive to the GI tract and must be taken with a full glass of water. The patient must then remain upright for at least 30 minutes to ensure that the drug has moved out of the esophagus and well into the GI system. Often, when a patient is admitted to a hospital or other health care facility, orders are written to continue drugs that were taken at home. There are often precautions, restrictions, or routines that the patient followed at home that don't fit into the facility's routine. In giving bisphosphonates in these settings, it's often difficult to ensure that a patient will* *have a full glass of water to take the pill (because of fluid restrictions or tests) and that she'll be able to take the drug on an empty stomach and remain upright for at least 30 minutes (because of test preparation, transportation, or physical condition).*

The Institute for Safe Medication Practices has reported several similar cases in the past 2 years. It recommends that when a patient who's taking Fosamax is admitted to the hospital, the drug be stopped during hospitalization to avoid this type of complication. Because Fosamax is now available in a once-a-week preparation, the patient may be able to switch to that form during hospitalization, making sure that the other cautions are heeded. On busy hospital floors, nurses might be more likely to provide these medications once a week rather than every day. With the large number of new drugs and drug preparations that are made available each year and the current shortage of nursing staff to tend to hospitalized patients, it's often difficult for a busy nurse to keep abreast of the specific details of each drug's administration. Patients who have been taking the drugs at home and are familiar with them are often a valuable resource, alerting the nurse when a specific drug may need to be researched before it's administered. When in doubt, check it out.

Missed doses

Catching up on missed doses of drugs requires special care. If a patient is away from his room for tests when medications are passed out, if an emergency in the unit results in the morning medications being passed out in the afternoon, or if a patient is allowed nothing to eat or drink because of upcoming tests and doesn't receive any medications for 1 day, the nurse has to decide if the patient can skip a dose or needs to take two doses at once.

Many drugs have special instructions about how to make up missed doses; some can be taken as soon as the patient realizes he missed a dose or when he returns from tests and is able to take the drug. The timing of the next dose depends on the drug. Certain drugs have precautions of a maximum dose for each day, and it's important that the patient not exceed that dose by doubling up on missed doses. Some drugs can be taken at the regularly scheduled time once a dose is made up.

Always check the drug guide when trying to determine how to make up a missed drug. Each drug is different, and the only way to be sure is to look it up. Perhaps the most complex drug timings for missed doses involve contraceptives (oral, vaginal ring, and patch forms). Give a woman using these contraceptives detailed instructions about what to do if she misses a dose, forgets or loses the vaginal ring, or the patch falls off.

PREVENT IT

Medication error: *Janelle, a 24-year-old graduate student, was prescribed Yasmin as an oral contraceptive. She took the pill for several months and then, during finals week, realized that she had missed a pill. Panicked, she took two pills and then, a few hours later, another pill "just to be sure." Three months later, she was seen in the University Health Service with symptoms that were related to a first-trimester pregnancy. Janelle was distraught and recalled the skipped pill. She told the staff that she was sure she was only supposed to take two pills the next day if she missed a dose.*

Prevention: *The staff was supportive of Janelle and inquired about where she got the information about the missed pills. She couldn't remember, but was sure she had learned that. She hadn't used another form of contraception during the days after the skipped pill — a point that's often stressed with missed pills. The staff retrieved a package insert from the*

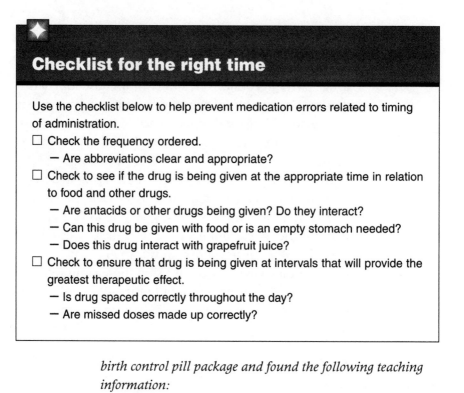

✦

Checklist for the right time

Use the checklist below to help prevent medication errors related to timing of administration.

☐ Check the frequency ordered.
  — Are abbreviations clear and appropriate?
☐ Check to see if the drug is being given at the appropriate time in relation to food and other drugs.
  — Are antacids or other drugs being given? Do they interact?
  — Can this drug be given with food or is an empty stomach needed?
  — Does this drug interact with grapefruit juice?
☐ Check to ensure that drug is being given at intervals that will provide the greatest therapeutic effect.
  — Is drug spaced correctly throughout the day?
  — Are missed doses made up correctly?

birth control pill package and found the following teaching information:

"If you miss one yellow pill, take that pill as soon as you remember it. If you miss two yellow pills in a row during week one or two, take two pills the day you remember and two pills the next day, then continue to take one a day until you have finished the package. Use another form of contraception during this time. If you miss two or three yellow pills in a row during week three, throw out that package and start a new one, taking one pill each day. You should use another form of contraception for the next 7 to 10 days. If you miss a white pill, continue taking the pills on the days designated and start the new package as usual."

Janelle said this information was ridiculous and that no one could possibly remember it all, especially if she was stressed from missing a pill. The staff encouraged her in the future to cut out the teaching information and paste it onto a card, which she could leave in a convenient place for easy reference should this happen again. They also advised Janelle to *use a backup method of contraception if she missed a dose to be safe. The staff used this experience as a stimulus for an education program about teaching students to use contraceptive pills effectively. They found that many preparations prescribed at the Health Service had unique and subtle differences in the way missed doses were handled. They made a file of that information for easy access if a patient called for help. The main thing to remember when a patient calls is "when in doubt, check it out."*

✦ Replay: The fifth right

The fifth right in the commonsense approach to preventing medication errors is to make sure that the time is right for giving the drug. This means ensuring that the timing ordered for doses of the drug has been interpreted correctly, that the time the drug is to be given doesn't create a conflict with another drug or food, and that the drug is actually delivered within the time frame that will provide its greatest therapeutic effect. This can be a great challenge for nurses in busy health care facilities. It's also challenging for the patient who's managing a complicated medical regimen at home. (See *Checklist for the right time*.)

Chapter

Righting the wrong

Medication errors occur every day. The combination of the national shortage of nurses and pharmacists, newer prescription drugs, and an increasing and aging population taking more drugs has provided additional opportunities for medication errors to occur. The overworked nurse or pharmacist can more easily make mistakes and won't have the time to double-check and carefully monitor patients. Fewer nurses and pharmacists means less time spent in actual patient teaching and more reliance on preprinted forms that may not give the patient the information he needs in a way he can understand it. This can lead to more errors for the patient who's unable to follow a drug regimen at home. Added to the increasing number of available drugs is the increasing consumer use of herbal medicines and alternative therapies, with their potential for interactions. In addition, patients have much easier access to drug information on the Internet and through direct-to-consumer advertising and are now demanding specific drugs for their treatment.

Each time an error is made, the time spent reporting the incident, monitoring and perhaps treating the patient, and providing education that can help prevent such errors from recurring, can severely challenge an already overburdened staff. Detecting and addressing medication errors takes time away from patient care and may create tension and distraction for the individual responsible for the error. These burdens, in turn, can have a snowball effect, setting the stage for future errors.

Numerous individuals and groups are at some level responsible for medication errors and must be part of the solution. The Food and Drug Administration (FDA), the Institute for Safe Medication Practices (ISMP), and several consumer groups are working together to decrease the incidence of medication errors; however, nurses are in a unique position to make a significant contribution to reducing such errors.

✦ Scope and source of the problem

In late 2001, a national study revealed that medication errors cost an estimated 76.6 to 136 billion dollars annually. The study defined a medication error as any preventable event that causes or leads to inappropriate medication use or patient harm while the medication is in the control of a health care professional, patient, or consumer.

The 5,366 medication errors tallied in the study involved problems with prescribing, labeling, packaging, dispensing, administering, and using drugs as well as problems with discussions and education about drug use. The researchers found that the most common error was the administration of the wrong dose of a drug to a patient (41%); second was the administration of the wrong drug to a patient (16%); and third was the administration of the drug by the wrong route (9.5%).

In evaluating the cause of the errors, researchers found that 65% involved the human factor. Human factors were defined as knowledge or performance deficits on the part of the prescriber, pharmacist, nurse, or patient that resulted in inaccurate calculations, inappropriate administration technique, failure to correctly identify the drug or the patient, and failure to administer the drug within the correct time frame. The second most common cause of errors was communication problems, such as poor handwriting and misunderstood verbal orders. In other words, errors occurred when the wrong drug was given to the wrong patient at the wrong dose by the wrong route and at the wrong time.

A problem of such magnitude must be addressed. While the media frequently points to the shortage of nurses and pharmacists as the chief culprit in medication errors, lack of manpower is but one of a number of factors.

✦ Historical perspective

Medication errors are an age-old problem. Although Florence Nightingale didn't mention the use of medications until the last few pages of her book, *Notes on Nursing,* published in 1859, her discussion of the subject offers evidence that medication errors were a thorny issue even in the early days of the nursing profession. She noted, for instance, that patients who didn't take the time to learn the names and components of their medications confused drugs with like-sounding names (colocynth and colchicum). This failure, according to Nightingale, amounted to "playing with sharp-edged tools with a vengeance." She also described patients who received drugs from their physicians and then shared them with neighbors who seemed to need these drugs, even though they didn't know their "exact and proper application and consequences."

In Nightingale's time, the best solution to medication errors was to ensure that only physicians prescribed and administered drugs. Nurses weren't even permitted to teach about drugs; that, too, was the physician's job. However, probably little teaching took place because teaching about pathology and drugs was seen as potentially causing more problems than it might solve. Thus, Nightingale's basic position was that the nurse didn't give drugs to herself or to others but, in the interest of safety, sent for the physician every time medication appeared to be needed.

Finding solutions

Nursing has come a long way since 1859, and the vast array of drugs used today to treat an equally vast number of disorders makes it impossible to send for the physician every time a drug is needed. The problems that Nightingale described, however — sound-alike and look-alike names causing confusion and the inappropriate use of drugs without an understanding of the consequences — remain problems today.

What's different now is that education is no longer perceived as a cause of medication errors, but rather is seen as key to their prevention. Today, it's widely believed that the more people know and understand about drugs and drug regimens, the safer their use of those drugs will be. However, education is just one component of the solution. Several efforts have been targeted toward using technology to decrease the possibility of error in the drug order and delivery process.

✦ Computerized order entry

The most easily addressed medication errors involve illegible handwriting, incorrect dosing as a result of misplaced or misread decimal points, and omission of information or failure to heed information about drug allergies or important drug-drug interactions. Computer systems to address these types of errors have been developed; one is the Computer Physician Order Entry

(CPOE) system. To use such systems, the physician enters an order directly into a computer rather than on
paper, thus eliminating the risk of errors in transcription or problems arising from illegible handwriting.
The computer system integrates the information from
the drug order with the patient's file, checking for allergies, other drugs the patient is using, and the patient's laboratory values. This quick, efficient checking
system then sends prompts to the physician questioning the appropriateness of the drug, the dosage, or another factor for that particular patient.

These systems promise to prevent many medication
errors now associated with poor handwriting, absent
allergy and interaction information, and failure to spot
precarious laboratory values.

IT'S A FACT

*In early 2002, an estimated 2% of the nation's hospitals were
using such systems. These hospitals have reported dramatic
decreases in the incidence of common medication errors.*

Snags in the system

Like all systems, computers can fail when the user isn't
properly oriented to the system or is too busy or
stressed to be alert. There have been reports of physicians not closing a patient's file, ordering the wrong
drug for a patient, selecting the wrong drug from a list,
or misspelling the patient's name and thereby ordering
drugs for a different patient. To compound this problem, patients may also be seeing more than one health
care provider. All providers may not have all of a patient's information in their systems, and the patient
may discuss with one physician that he's using over-

the-counter (OTC) drugs or alternative therapies that could interfere or interact with his medical treatment, yet fail to mention it to another.

Sometimes the programs themselves are problematic. In 2002, the ISMP reported that while one computer system was found to automatically round up dosages, others used a naked decimal point routinely, confusing prescribing issues.

However, computer systems offer good, quick checks on the information that's available, and some analysts believe that, as better systems become available, computer use may become the standard.

✦ Computer pharmacy programs

Computer programs are also used in pharmacies to alert the pharmacist to the potential for drug-drug interactions, to the existence of a patient's drug allergies, or to an inappropriate dose selection for a drug. These programs have had some success, but they aren't perfect. In the end, as with CPOE systems, the accuracy of these programs depends on the accuracy of the person using the program.

✦ Raising awareness

Standardized medication error reporting systems have streamlined the process of reporting errors to a central source for evaluation and alerts. These systems may have led to the media's fascination with medication errors. In truth, the errors have been occurring all along, but an adequate reporting system didn't exist.

Use of these reporting systems has focused attention on the types of medication errors and alerted health care providers and the drug industry to be more mindful of potential errors — confusing drug names, confusing packaging, and inadequate education programs.

Furthermore, this has contributed to the institution of new FDA regulations for naming new drugs, packaging changes to reduce the incidence of mistakes between look-alike names and packages, and more appropriate teaching literature regarding drug administration and drug information for consumers.

New naming and labeling guidelines

Each new study of medication errors seems to produce more alarming statistics. One study carried out by the FDA in 2002 found that:

✦ 48% of medication errors related to the wrong dose being given (errors in communication, reading, and calculating)
✦ 17% related to the wrong route being used (communication errors, incorrect technique)
✦ 16% related to the wrong drug being given (communication and handwriting problems, confusion between look-alike and sound-alike drug names)
✦ 8% related to the wrong timing of the dose
✦ 3% were related to the wrong patient
✦ 8% were unclassifiable and listed as "other." (See *FDA study findings.*)

After reviewing the causes, the FDA felt that it could most effectively address mistakes related to administering the wrong drug. More than 1,000 drugs have similar names that are easily confused.

IT'S A FACT

A patient with diabetes died when his prescription for chlorpropamide (an antidiabetic agent) was inadvertently filled with chlorpromazine (an antianxiety agent). Under the new guidelines, the labels of these two drugs should appear as chlorproMAZINE and chlorproPAMIDE. The use of small and capital letters in the label should alert the person dis-

FDA study findings

In early 2002, the Food and Drug Administration (FDA) reported the results of a 2001 survey on medication errors. It estimated that nearly 1.3 million Americans experience a medication error each year.

Medication errors

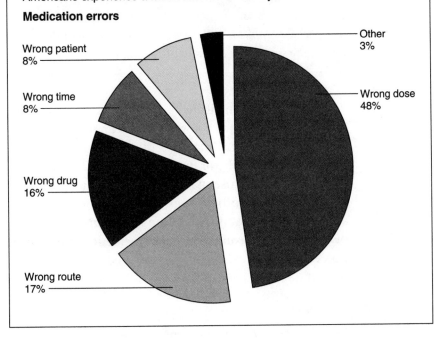

Other
3%

Wrong patient
8%

Wrong time
8%

Wrong dose
48%

Wrong drug
16%

Wrong route
17%

pensing or administering the medications to the potential name confusion.

To avoid errors due to sound-alike or look-alike drug names, the FDA established new guidelines for labeling such drugs. Letters sent to manufacturers of the most commonly confused drugs requested that labels be changed to avoid future confusion. The use of different colors, different type fonts, and different-sized letters in the revised labels could alert the health care provider to and help him distinguish between confusing names.

IT'S A FACT

Lamictal (lamotrigine) is used to treat epilepsy, and Lamisil (terbinafine) is an antifungal drug. Although the FDA issued three warnings in 3 years about possible confusion between these two drugs, three people reportedly experienced serious seizures due to a mix-up. Under the new labeling suggestions, the label for Lamictal will appear as LAMictal with the first part of the name in a different color than the rest.

The FDA also established a volunteer group to test potential drug names before a drug is approved for marketing. Since the inception of this committee, almost one third of the brand names suggested have been rejected because of the possibility that they could be confused with other drugs. The FDA hopes that by addressing the root of one of the most common causes of error — name confusion — the incidence of medication errors will be dramatically reduced.

Consumer education

Many groups such as the American Association for Retired Persons (AARP) are focusing efforts on consumer education about drugs and drug usage. National media campaigns concerning the accurate reading of drug labels have been launched. Web sites have been designed to help patients understand what they need to know about their drugs, what questions to ask, and when to be cautious about OTC or herbal therapy use.

✦ The nurse's role

As important as all these strategies are, the fact is that alert, educated, and responsible individuals ultimately prevent medication errors. Technology, for instance, can only go so far. Computers aren't foolproof; mistakes can happen if they aren't programmed or used correctly. On a more human level, warning stickers can fall off, people can forget to check interaction precautions, and patients can forget drug names, dosage times, and adverse incidents. The alert, critically thinking, questioning person is the only reliable defense against medication errors.

While it clearly isn't her sole responsibility, the nurse is most commonly the last step between the patient and the drug—whether the nurse is administering the drug or teaching the patient about self-administration. The vigilance of every health care provider may be the best safeguard against errors, yet the nurse is often the ultimate deterrent.

Reinforce the "right" way

The underlying rationale for safe nursing drug administration has always been the five "rights"—the right patient, the right drug, the right dose, the right route, and the right time for administration. When a medication error occurs, it involves one of these five issues.

Medication errors can be prevented in clinical practice by maintaining regular checks on these rights. However, checking the rights doesn't simply mean verifying that you're giving the right patient the right dose of the right drug by the right route at the right time; it involves thoughtful checks of the finer points. As with other practices that become routine, administering medications can become a series of automatically performed steps. Over time, the fine points of ensuring patient safety can be overlooked.

A periodic review of the basics for checking the five rights should become standard for all practicing nurses. Post a list in the medicine room, on the medication cart, or in the front of the drug guide. (See *Checklist for preventing medication errors.*) In today's fast-paced world with staffing shortages, sicker patients, and myriad new and changing drugs, no one can be too careful when it comes to patient safety and preventing medication errors.

When in doubt, check it out

The basic rule that all nurses can adopt to help ensure the safety of drug therapy and to prevent medication errors is simple: "When in doubt, check it out." Never assume that you know all the drugs, all the drug effects, all the dosages, all the routes, and all of the timing complications. Drug therapy — indications, dosages, warnings, and routes — changes daily. If something doesn't look familiar, seems illogical, or just doesn't seem right, look it up, ask someone else, and check it out. Feel confident that the right drug is given to the right patient at the right dose by the right route and at the right time. Don't feel uncomfortable about questioning a drug order or clarifying an indication — the nurse who administers the drug is ultimately responsible for proper administration of a drug.

Red flags

The ISMP recently published a list of phrases that, if heard, should raise a warning about patient safety and prompt further investigation into the situation.

✦ *"That's what the doctor ordered."* This may indicate that the nurse doesn't know about a specific drug, doesn't have time to check it out, or doesn't want to be bothered.

✦ *"The doctor told me to do it that way."* This suggests that the nurse has her own routine and doesn't appreciate being questioned, but feels safe placing responsibility with the physician.

Checklist for preventing medication errors

RIGHT PATIENT

☐ Check the patient's identification.
☐ Check the patient's medication history. (Does he have drug allergies? Does he use over-the-counter agents, herbal preparations, daily medications, or other prescription drugs?)
☐ Check the patient's pregnancy status, if applicable.

RIGHT DRUG

☐ Check the generic name, brand name, and intended indication of pre-scribed medications (during preparation and right before administration).
☐ Check to see if medications have been stored and prepared properly and if they make sense for the patient.

RIGHT DOSE

☐ Check the prescriber's order for clarity. Watch out for decimal points; zeros; abbreviations; and run-together, sound-alike, and look-alike words.
☐ Check to see if the drug dosage ordered makes sense for the patient. (Is the patient at extremes for age, weight, and renal or liver function?)
☐ Check to see if the drug dosage ordered is accurate. (Are mathematical calculations correct? Do you need to administer more than two or three standard units of the drug? Is the medication allowed to be cut if necessary?)

RIGHT ROUTE

☐ Check the route ordered. (Are abbreviations clear and appropriate? Is the drug available in the form that it has been ordered? Can the patient take the drug by the route ordered?)
☐ Check that you remember the correct administration technique for the route ordered.

RIGHT TIME

☐ Check the frequency ordered. (Are abbreviations clear and appropriate?)
☐ Check to see if the drug is being given at the appropriate time in relation to food and other medications.
☐ Check to make sure that the drug is being given at intervals that will provide the greatest therapeutic effects.

✦ *"The patient says that's what he does at home."* This may indicate that the nurse doesn't know what to do and is placing responsibility with the patient, or that the patient had other ideas and the nurse didn't have the time or energy to argue otherwise.

✦ *"This dosage was published in AJN in November as the right thing to order."* Be cautious of those who answer questions with citations of scholarly works. When challenged, some people respond this way to avoid an unpleasant confrontation. They may even make up the citation. Ask to see the journal.

✦ *"This is a special case."* If the case was special, the unit would be aware of it. This is a frequent excuse when someone hasn't taken the time to get further information.

✦ *"The patient is on a protocol."* This could be a legitimate response; however, if a special protocol was being used, the unit would have that fact posted to prevent any violation of the protocol. Ask to see the protocol.

✦ *"We always do it that way."* That may be the case, but it doesn't necessarily make it the *right* way. Remember the traveling nurse in chapter 6 who always crushed the medications of nursing home patients? Some of those medications were ones that shouldn't be crushed.

Never accept an excuse when you question an order or a policy. When in doubt, always check it out yourself. Remember, the nurse who gives the medication is responsible for her actions.

Nursing shortage as a benefit

The national nursing shortage continues. To overcome this, many nurses are floated to work in unfamiliar units and many facilities hire temporary help from traveling nurse groups or nursing agencies. As a result, nurses in such situations may not be familiar with their new unit or facility's routine and, therefore, may raise some questions.

This isn't necessarily a bad thing. Nurses need to question policy and routine to keep it fresh and clinically appropriate; new staff members may offer insights to a problem that aren't apparent to the regular staff or may suggest new ways to improve patient care. However, a negative effect can result when the outside nurse doesn't follow procedure, introduces a new procedure that's against policy, or doesn't ask questions when she should. Nurses need to be responsible and accountable for their actions.

Keep good records

The patient's chart is a legal document. "If it isn't documented, it didn't happen" is a critical teaching point for new staff and a wise reminder for experienced staff. Before health care facilities are accredited, there's a flurry of activity to ensure that all records are in order and that the staff understands and follows facility policies.

The patient chart is the only way that health care providers can track the details and events of the patient's care, such as when drugs were given, patient responses, and any problems that occurred. It's how the next shift provides continuity of care. As with other routine practices, documentation should be periodically reviewed before a problem occurs that requires an incident report.

Paperwork is the bane of most busy health care professionals. The shift may end, only to be followed by hours of paperwork to document the day's events. Because documentation is a time-consuming activity and because it doesn't appear to be actual patient care, many nurses use shortcuts for completing their paperwork. Standardized care plans or flowsheets with checklists eliminate the need to write explanations and are often used in busy facilities. A nursing student may learn in the classroom that before an antihypertensive drug is given, she should check the patient's blood pressure and document it in the chart. After the first week as a graduate nurse taking care of several patients, she may find herself skipping that step. Is it more important to make sure that the patient gets the drug or to assess and document what's going on with the patient? Most nurses are forced to select the former—to make sure that the drugs are administered as ordered and worry about the fine points later. Some nurses even sign for all of the medications they're going to give before they actually give them because the medication record is available, they don't want to have to go through the list again, and they're confident that they'll be giving the drugs. However, events happen during a shift. Remember the patient in chapter 6 who hid his sleeping pills in the pillowcase? Legally, drugs should be signed for only after they have been administered; by signing for the drugs, you're verifying the patient identity, drug, dose, route, and time on the patient record.

Report any errors

Nurses are often in the best position to observe potential or actual medication errors. Although facilities have internal error-reporting policies to protect staff and patients and to identify the need for educational programs, it's also important to submit information about errors to national programs. These national programs, coordinated by the United States Pharmacopeia (USP), help gather and disseminate information about medication errors to prevent repetition at other sites by other providers.

The reporting of actual or potential errors results in alerts and publicity about issues such as sound-alike drug names, problems with abbreviations, the need for clear writing of dosages and times, incorrect calculations, and transcribing issues. The reports might also result in the issuing of prescriber warnings to alert health care providers of actual or potential medication errors and prevent recurrence of these errors. For example, after several reports of confusion between amrinone and amiodarone, the FDA recommended that the manufacturer of amrinone change the drug name from amrinone to inamrinone. If someone hadn't reported the confusion, assuming that the problem had occurred only at his facility, the name change wouldn't have taken place and many more patients might have suffered. The listing of sound-alike and look-alike names on page 105 was compiled from reports from across the country.

If you observe or participate in an actual or potential medication error, it's important to report that error to the national clearinghouse to benefit other health care professionals. To streamline the reporting process and simplify participation by professionals, the USP maintains a central reporting center from which it disseminates information to the FDA, drug manufacturers, and the ISMP. An actual or potential error can be reported by calling *1-800-23-ERROR,* the USP Medication Errors Reporting Program. Its office will send a pre-addressed mailer to complete and return. Alternatively, its Web site, *www.usp.org,* allows anyone to report an error on-line or print the reporting form to mail or fax to the USP. The person reporting an error may remain anonymous to all facilities to which the report will be sent if he's uncomfortable sharing the information openly. Errors may also be reported to the USP through the ISMP web site at *www.ismp.org.* This site also offers a discussion forum on medication errors.

Reportable problems

Errors (or potential errors) involving the administration of the wrong drug, strength, or dose of a drug; incorrect routes of administration; miscalculations; misuse of medical equipment; mistakes in prescribing or transcribing (misunderstanding of verbal orders); or errors resulting from sound-alike or look-alike names should be reported. When reporting one of these, the following information will be required:

✦ a description of the error or preventable adverse drug reaction (What went wrong?)

✦ if this was an actual medication accident (did it reach the patient) or an error that was discovered before it reached the patient

✦ patient outcome (Did the patient suffer any adverse effects?)

✦ type of practice site (hospital, private office, retail pharmacy, drug company, long-term care facility)

✦ generic name of all products involved

✦ trade (brand) name of all products involved

✦ dosage form, concentration, or strength

✦ if the error was based on miscommunication (Is a copy of the order available? Are package label samples or pictures available, if requested?)

✦ recommendations for error prevention.

The reporting individual will also need to provide his name, title, facility address, e-mail, and fax or telephone numbers in case there's a need for additional details.

The ISMP publishes case studies and publicizes warnings and alerts based on clinician reports of medication errors. Its efforts have helped to increase the recognition of many types of errors. To check for updated alerts, warnings, and related links, visit the USP at *www.usp.org*, the ISMP at *www.ismp.org*, or the FDA warnings section at *www.fda.gov*.

Become educated

Education is key to the prevention of medication errors. However, staff education is often left to the inservice or continuing education department or the individual nurse who's giving the drug. Drug companies need to be more involved.

Make sure that an up-to-date drug guide is easily accessible at work. Make a note of convenient Web sites to access when time allows. Share the information among colleagues. If all nurses in a unit shared information on new drugs, indications, warnings, or refreshers on administration techniques, an entire year of staff education programs could result. Post helpful notices, tables, or charts in an area where other people can also benefit from them. When a list of drugs that shouldn't be cut, crushed, or chewed was distributed during morning rounds at a home health agency, two nurses reported back that they had used the information and prevented potential drug problems that same day. Neither nurse was aware of the problems with altering drugs until someone read an article, made a copy of the list, and shared that information.

Stay educated

Getting educated isn't enough. Prevention of medication errors depends upon nurses to continually brush up on their skills and keep their knowledge and technique current.

To get through the busy day, most nurses find it helpful to establish a routine and then follow it. However, several studies have shown that routine itself leads to a blurring of details, rationale, and protocol. When nurses and patients get into a routine, they eventually think that what they're doing is what they were taught. A periodic review of the five rights, administration techniques, key timing factors for drug therapy, and the newest drugs on the market should become the subjects of regular refresher courses — courses as significant as the annual cardiopulmonary resuscitation certification. Recognizing that it's human nature to forget, the education department should encourage attendance at refresher programs, and nurses shouldn't regard attendance requests as punishment.

Educate the patient

Another critical part of preventing medication errors, and often the most neglected area of health care, is patient education. Busy units or offices, crowded pharmacies, and hurried patients often discourage individual teaching. Many states require that pharmacies provide written information about each drug dispensed to patients. Often, this written information — which may contain words that seem technical or unfamiliar to the patient — is stapled to the prescription bag with the assumption that the patient will read and understand it. But in June 2002, the FDA released results of a national study that revealed that while 89% of patients received the information, less than 50% read the information or found it useful. A large pharmacy chain, short on pharmacists and extremely busy, meets state requirements by having each patient sign for his prescription when picking it up. Unknown to the patient, he's also signing a form attesting that he refused a personal consultation with the pharmacist. Legally, the pharmacy is covered;it has a signed statement from the patient dismissing a discussion that could have improved his medical regimen and prevented problems.

The patient is the last in the series of crosschecks to prevent medication errors. The prescriber, pharmacist, and nurse may miss something in the chain of events that occur during the ordering, dispensing, and administering of a drug. However, the medical regimen of each patient is unique to that patient. The patient must understand it so that he can be his own best advocate.

PREVENT IT

Medication error: A patient in the oncologist's office was told that she would receive methotrexate (Folex) I.V., followed an hour later by fluorouracil (5-FU) I.V. The oncologist explained that the methotrexate could be toxic and that he was going to order a leucovorin rescue (Wellcovorin) to be started 24 hours after the methotrexate. He wrote an order for leucovorin 25 mg P.O. one every 6 hours for 6 doses starting 24 hours after chemotherapy. The patient took the prescription to the pharmacy, where the pharmacist wrote the following on the label: Take one tablet every 6 hours for 6 days starting 24 hours before the chemotherapy. When the patient got home and read the label on the bottle, she became concerned that these instructions were different from what her physician had stated. She called the clinic to verify the order. Luckily, the patient had heard the physician's instructions correctly. If she had followed the label instructions, she wouldn't have had the benefit of the leucovorin rescue and could have become ill from the chemotherapy.

Prevention: This medication error was prevented because the regimen had been explained to the patient. When the patient was confused about the labeling on the drug, she was comfortable checking with her physician. If this patient hadn't received individual teaching, the error wouldn't have been caught and she could have experienced serious toxic effects. Taking the time to provide teaching saved time, money, and patient suffering in this case.

A 2001 survey of health practices revealed that fewer than half of all patients actually take their medications correctly. That same survey estimated that this lack of knowledge may increase the cost of health care by more than 73 billion dollars. Thus, patient education should become a priority for all health care facilities, not only to save money but also to improve the care and welfare of their patients.

Although many nursing programs don't include formal training in patient education, nurses are assumed to be the best health teachers. However, patient education isn't as simple as it might seem. A survey of new parents who were also college graduates revealed that many couldn't interpret the labels on OTC cold or allergy bottles or they couldn't determine the ingredients or the dosage that should be given to their children. (See *Survey on OTC drug use.*) In fact, research has shown that when it comes to health care, almost one-half of the adult population in the United States can be assumed to be functionally illiterate. Written brochures or standardized printouts may be of no use, especially if they contain large or technical words.

People who have difficulty reading learn to hide their problem. They may get through their lives without anyone recognizing that they can't read or understand simple orders or signs. Identifying reading problems isn't easy; first, you have to be looking for the problem. A survey of graduating nursing students revealed that most of them assumed that all patients could read. Research shows that the average nonmedical person who reads medical information comprehends information that's written at the fifth grade level. Imagine attending a nuclear engineering conference. As the keynote address is being given, you sit there and have no idea what's going on, while the rest of the audience appears to follow what's being said. Many patients feel that way each time a physician or nurse explains a procedure, drug, or medical regimen.

Survey on OTC drug use

In 2002, the National Council on Patient Information and Education published the results of a national survey done by Harris Interactive in 2001 regarding the use of over-the-counter (OTC) drugs. The survey was prompted by reports that over 100,000 OTC drug products with more than 1,000 active ingredients are currently available. Over 700 of these OTC products contain ingredients that were available only by prescription less than 30 years ago.

Most of the people surveyed (more than three out of five) reported routine use of OTC products; however, only 34% could identify the active ingredient in their OTC drug. Although 95% of respondents reported reading a portion of the OTC drug label, they were selective in what they read. Forty-one percent stated that they read the label to find out the use of the drug, the symptoms it would treat, and the recommended dosage. Only one in three looked for the name of the active ingredient, and only one in five actually read label warnings.

MISGUIDED OVERDOSING

Because so many people have limited knowledge about the OTC drugs that they use, it isn't surprising that over 69% report taking more than the recommended dose of a drug (reasoning that if one is good, two is better; forgetting when the next dose is due; taking the drug when the symptoms return regardless of time). Over 35% of responders said that they're very likely to combine OTC and prescription drugs when they have multiple symptoms.

This survey supports health care providers' concerns about patients inadvertently taking too much of an active ingredient and developing toxic levels; about OTC drug use causing drug-drug interactions with prescription drugs; and about the chronic use of OTC drugs masking the symptoms of potentially serious underlying medical conditions.

The survey results were released to coincide with a national effort to educate consumers. "BeMedWise" is a television campaign designed to raise consumer awareness about OTC drug use, the possibility of inadvertent drug overdose, and the importance of reading and understanding drug labels. The complete survey is available for review at *www.bemdewise.org*.

No one wants to appear stupid. Would you feel comfortable raising your hand and asking the keynote speaker what on earth he was talking about? Similarly, most patients won't interrupt or ask questions.

Compound that confusion with the stress caused by concern and fear about their health. How will this affect their budget? How will this drug regimen fit into their day? How will they get to the drug store? Are they ready to be discharged? These concerns may be more pressing to the patient than learning how a take the medication correctly. Also, remember that because the patient is feeling ill, he may not be able to focus or concentrate on the instructions. Thus, patients who receive drug information are in the precarious position of being dependent on the prescriber, which makes your job as an educator all the more important.

Guidelines for teaching
Face-to-face, verbal communication is key to having the information understood. When relaying information, remember to keep it simple.

+ *Offer information in small amounts.* Patients are much more likely to comprehend only the information they perceive to be pertinent to them and dismiss the rest. Although health care providers want patients to understand the reason for their condition and its underlying physiology, patients may simply want to know what the interventions are. Tell the patient:
  - the name of the drug (essential when a patient sees other health care providers or travels out of the area)
  - the dose of the drug (say "two tablets" rather than using measurements such as milligrams or units, which may diminish the patient's focus)
  - when to take the drug (for most people, specifying a time is important; telling them they have to

take two pills four times a day may translate to
taking eight pills between 8 a.m. and noon)
- what to expect (dizziness, drowsiness, frequent
  bathroom use, other effects that may affect their
  daily activities)
- any special precautions (such as, don't mix with
  grapefruit juice, or call if you have bloody diarrhea).

✦ *Provide written information as a back-up reference for
  the patient to take home.* Simply handing a patient
  written information isn't teaching. Are you sure
  the patient can read? Does he understand the
  words that are used? Is he interpreting the information correctly? Information should be written
  to be understood by individuals at the fifth grade
  level. To avoid overwhelming the patient, present
  key information in lists or bulleted points rather
  than long paragraphs. Use simple diagrams or pictures to illustrate a technique, such as how to apply eye drops, and highlight only critical information — for example, the number to call if there's a
  problem or question.

✦ *Follow up.* Make sure that the patient has understood all teaching by asking him to repeat the information. Ask open-ended questions; don't ask
  questions that can be answered "yes" or "no" because the patient has a 50% chance of being correct despite not knowing the answer. Ask the patient to demonstrate the technique rather than
  asking him if he's performing it correctly. Provide
  extensive follow-up. A patient who has been using a nebulizer for 10 years may have developed
  bad habits or forgotten how to hold the nebulizer
  or position his head correctly because it's routine.

✦ *Maintain a positive attitude.* Despite being busy, being frustrated with the schedule, or having col-

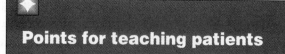

Points for teaching patients

Use the following guide as a reminder of the points you should cover when teaching a patient about medications:
✦ drug name, dosage, and action
✦ timing of administration
✦ special storage and preparation information
✦ specific over-the-counter drugs and herbal or alternative therapies to avoid
✦ special comfort measures
✦ safety measures that need to be observed
✦ adverse effects to report to health care provider
✦ warnings about drug toxicity
✦ reminders to keep the drug out of the reach of children.

leagues or patient's relatives present demands, take a deep breath and present the needed information to the patient in an upbeat manner. Doing so will prevent the patient from feeling stupid. Relate to the patient that the teaching contains important information and that he's a valuable and respected member of the team managing his health care. The patient may then retain the information and may feel comfortable in calling with questions or for additional information. (See *Points for teaching patients.*)

If a certain drug regimen is used frequently in a particular unit, it may be helpful to print individual teaching sheets. Patients who have used the drug may also be helpful to someone just starting a particular drug. Sometimes, health care professionals forget that certain words may be foreign to a layperson. For example, *edema* is a common term in medicine, but patients who link edema with swelling may have difficulty relating swelling in the skin to problems with the heart or vascular system. A patient who has had experience with a drug may shed a different perspective on how to present information about that drug.

IT'S A FACT

In March 1997, to improve consumer safety, the FDA passed a regulation that set guidelines for labeling OTC drugs. These guidelines advocate the use of language that's understandable and print that's readable so that it's easier for consumers to read and understand the OTC drug label. As of May 2002, most OTC drugs must conform to these new labeling standards.

✦ Replay: The five rights

It's estimated that nearly 1.3 million Americans experience a medication error each year. These errors are costly in terms of time and money. A collaborated effort to improve staff and patient education, to continually update and refine skills, to report problems in an effort to prevent problems, and to improve the process by which medications are ordered, dispensed, and administered is needed. The five rights — making sure the right patient receives the right drug at the right dose by the right route at the route time — are the health care worker's best defense against this growing problem. Use them well.

Appendices and index

Appendix A
Antidotes for poisoning and overdose

Specific antidotes react chemically with, or block the receptor sites of, specific toxins. This chemical reaction decreases the toxic effects and, in many situations, reverses the effects of the poison or overdose. Generally, there are no contraindications for the use of antidotes; they're used only in potentially serious situations when the benefits clearly outweigh the risks to the patient.

Before using an antidote, perform a patient assessment, including a careful history of the time and amount of the exposure to the toxin. Timing is usually crucial for treatment. When performing the patient's physical assessment, include vi-

GENERIC NAME	BRAND NAME	PURPOSE
acetylcysteine	Mucomyst, Mucosil, Parvolex	Antidote to prevent or lessen hepatic injury after acetaminophen overdose
atropine sulfate	(no brand name)	Treatment of anticholinesterase poisoning (organophosphorous insecticides); antidote for muscarine poisoning in mushroom poisoning
calcium chloride, calcium gluconate	(no brand name)	Antidote for overdose of calcium channel blockers
charcoal, activated	Actidose-Aqua, CharcoAid, Liqui-Char	Absorbs toxic substances from GI tract, inhibiting GI absorption; emergency treatment of poisoning by many chemicals and drugs, including acetaminophen and benzodiazepines

tal signs, orientation, and blood chemistries appropriate to the toxin and the antidote. Have supportive measures readily available, including life-support equipment, I.V. fluids to counteract shock, and ventilation devices.

When educating the patient and family, be sure to include reasons for the antidote, adverse effects to expect, and drugs and other products to avoid after use of the antidote. In cases of accidental overdose, work with the patient and family to determine ways to prevent this from happening in the future.

DOSAGE	NURSING MANAGEMENT
140 mg/kg P.O. as a loading dose, followed by 70 mg/kg every 4 hours after loading dose for a total of 17 doses; I.V. dose is available if oral route is impossible	Begin treatment within 24 hours of overdose. Empty stomach by gastric lavage; use activated charcoal if feasible to decrease the amount acetaminophen absorbed; obtain blood chemistries and acetaminophen levels prior to therapy and daily until levels are returned to nontoxic levels. Provide supportive care for electrolyte imbalances, hypoglycemia, and clotting problems related to hepatic injury.
2 to 3 mg I.V. repeated every 5 to 6 minutes until signs of atropine toxicity occur	Provide ventilatory support, cardiac massage as needed; monitor vital signs continually until stabilized.
4.6 to 16 mEq I.V.	Monitor vital signs continuously; monitor serum calcium levels; be prepared to provide life support and to counteract hypotension and bradycardia as appropriate.
30 to 100 g or 1 g/kg P.O. (5 to 10 times the amount of the toxin ingested)	Administer as soon as possible after ingestion. Induce emesis before giving activated charcoal; give to conscious patient only. Maintain life-support equipment on standby.

GENERIC NAME	BRAND NAME	PURPOSE
deferoxamine	Desferal	Antidote for acute or chronic iron toxicity
dexrazoxane	Zinecard	Reduction of incidence and severity of cardiotoxicity associated with doxorubicin therapy
digoxin immune fab	Digibind, DigiFab	Treatment of life-threatening digoxin intoxication or overdose
dimercaprol	BAL In Oil	Chelating agent; antidote for acute mercury poisoning; arsenic, gold, chronic mercury poisoning; lead poisoning in combination with edetate disodium
edetate calcium disodium, edetate disodium	Calcium Disodium Versenate, Endrate	Treatment of lead poisoning, calcium overdose, digoxin toxicity

DOSAGE	NURSING MANAGEMENT
Acute iron toxicity: 1 g I.M. followed by 0.5 g I.M. every 4 hours for two doses; then 0.5 g I.M. every 4 to 12 hours based on response. *Chronic iron toxicity:* 0.5 to 1 g I.M. daily	Monitor neurologic status during therapy; rash and pain at injection sites is common; stop drug and reevaluate if vision becomes impaired.
Dexrazoxane:doxorubicin ratio should be 10:1 I.V.	Administer by slow I.V. push or rapid I.V. drip; don't mix with other drugs; use special caution when handling and disposing of drug.
Dosage determined by serum digoxin level or amount of digoxin ingested; if this information can't be obtained, use 760 mg I.V. (20 vials)	Monitor serum digoxin prior to and periodically during therapy; monitor cardiac response continually; maintain life support equipment on standby at all times; don't redigitalize patient until drug has cleared the system, several days to 1 week. Teach patient to report palpitations, dizziness, and muscle cramps.
2.5 to 5 mg/kg I.M. every 4 to 6 hours I.M. for up to 10 days	Administer by deep I.M. injection only; monitor for severe nausea and vomiting, medication may be needed. Teach patient to report severe headache or weakness and tingling in the extremities.
Lead poisoning: Adult: 5 ml I.V. undiluted twice daily for up to 5 days or 35 mg/kg I.M. twice daily. *Pediatric:* 35 mg/kg I.M. twice daily for 3 to 5 days followed by a 2-day rest before repeating *Hypercalcemia or digoxin toxicity: Adult:* 50 mg/kg/day I.V. for 5 consecutive days then 2 free days followed by another series. *Pediatric:* 40 mg/kg/day I.V.	Prepare a schedule of rest and drug days; monitor electrolytes and blood urea nitrogen levels prior to and periodically during therapy; monitor cardiac rhythm if used to treat digoxin overdose. Teach patient to report pain at injection site or difficulty voiding.

GENERIC NAME	BRAND NAME	PURPOSE
flumazenil	Romazicon	Complete or partial reversal of benzodiazepine effects
glucagon	Glucagon Emergency Kit	Counteracts hypoglycemia from insulin overdose or insulin shock; natural hormone that accelerates the breakdown of glycogen to glucose
leucovorin calcium	Wellcovorin	Leucovorin "rescue" after high dose methotrexate therapy; reverses toxic effects of methotrexate on normal cells
mesna	Mesnex	Reacts chemically with urotoxic ifosfamide; used prophylactically to prevent hemorrhagic cystitis when ifosfamide is being used
methylene blue	Urolene Blue	Treatment for cyanide poisoning or nitrate poisoning; reduces hemeoglobin to hemoglobin
nalmefene, naloxone, naltrexone	Narcan, Revex, ReVia, Trexan	Narcotic antagonists; block opioid receptors and displace the opioid from the receptor

DOSAGE	NURSING MANAGEMENT
0.2 mg I.V., wait 45 seconds and repeat at 60-second intervals until response occurs, to a total dose of 1 mg. *Acute overdose:* 0.2 mg I.V., wait 30 seconds and repeat once with 0.3-mg dose I.V.; repeat with 0.5-mg doses to a total of 3 mg.	Inject into running I.V.; monitor clinical response and sedation carefully; have life-support equipment available; instruct patient to avoid over-the-counter drugs and alcohol for at least 18 to 24 hours after receiving this drug.
0.5 to 1 mg S.C., I.V., or I.M.; may repeat dose once or twice until response occurs	Monitor skin (for clamminess), color, orientation, and vital signs; obtain blood glucose levels and adjust dosage accordingly. Teach patient and family how to recognize signs of hypoglycemia and to administer glucagon S.C.
10 mg/m^2 P.O., I.M., or I.V. until methotrexate level falls below 5×10^{-8} M	Begin rescue within 24 hours of methotrexate administration. Arrange for fluid loading and urine alkalinization to decrease methotrexate toxicity; give drug orally if possible; maintain life-support equipment on standby.
20% of the ifosfamide dose given as a single I.V. dose at time of each ifosfamide injection and repeated at 4 and 8 hours	Prepare within 6 hours of use, discard unused portion; record times of injection to ensure accurate timing of dose; monitor patient for signs of hemorrhagic cystitis.
1 to 2 mg/kg I.V. injected over several minutes	Inject slowly over several minutes; avoid S.C. injection; monitor blood chemistries; monitor patient continuously, maintaining life support equipment on standby.
Nalmefene: 0.5 mg/70 kg I.V., then 1 mg/70 kg I.V. 2 to 5 minutes later; maximum dose, 1.5 mg/70 kg *Naloxone:* 0.4 to 2 mg I.V., S.C., or I.M.; may repeat at 2- to 3-minute intervals; maximum dose, 10 mg *Naltrexone:* used for maintenance program for narcotic withdrawal 50 mg/24 hours P.O.	Advise patient to avoid opiate-containing drugs, including analgesics and cough and cold preparations, for several weeks after taking this drug. Dizziness and drowsiness are common adverse reactions.

GENERIC NAME	BRAND NAME	PURPOSE
neostigmine methylsulfate	Prostigmin	Antidote for nondepolarizing neuromuscular junction blockers
penicillamine	Cuprimine, Depen	Chelating agent; forms inactive complex with copper, leading to rapid urinary excretion
physostigmine	Antilirium	Treatment of overdose of anticholinergics, including tricyclic antidepressants and diazepam overdose
pralidoxime chloride	Protopam Chloride	Antidote to poisoning due to organophosphate pesticides and chemicals with anticholinesterase activities
protamine sulfate	(no brand name)	Heparin antagonist; used to treat heparin overdose
pyridoxine hydrochloride	Aminoxin, Nestrex	Competitively blocks isoniazid (INH) effects in cases of INH toxicity
succimer	Chemet	Treatment of lead poisoning; chelates lead in the system
vitamin K (phytonadione)	Mephyton, AquaMEPHYTON	Treatment of prothrombin-induced deficiency caused by overdose of oral anticoagulants

DOSAGE	NURSING MANAGEMENT
0.5 to 2.5 mg I.V. by slow injection; repeat as needed; maximum dose, 5 mg	Administer 0.6 to 1.2 mg I.V. atropine before giving neostigmine. Monitor patient continually; maintain life-support equipment on standby.
1 g/day P.O., in divided doses four times daily; up to 2 g may be needed	Monitor patient carefully for potentially fatal myasthenic syndrome and bone marrow depression; arrange for blood chemistries prior to and at least every 2 weeks during therapy; administer drug on an empty stomach at least 30 to 60 minutes before meals and at least 2 hours after evening meal.
0.5 to 2 mg I.M. or I.V.	Administer I.V. slowly, ≤1 mg/minute; have atropine on standby in case of cholinergic crisis; monitor patient response carefully.
1 to 2 g I.V. as a 15- to 30-minute infusion; repeat in 1 hour, give additional doses as needed	Give as soon as possible after exposure. Give 2 to 4 mg atropine I.V. concomitantly with pralidoxime; maintain airway and have life-support equipment on standby, as needed.
Dose determined by heparin dose; 1 mg I.V. neutralizes 90 USP U heparin from lung sources or 115 USP U heparin from intestinal sources	Monitor coagulation studies to adjust dosage and to detect "heparin rebound" response to drug; maintain life-support equipment on standby.
4 g I.V. followed by 1 g I.M. every 30 minutes	Monitor injection sites for any sign of irritation; maintain life-support equipment on standby.
10 mg/kg P.O. every 8 hours for 5 days, then 10 mg/kg P.O. every 12 hours for 2 weeks	Obtain serum lead levels prior to therapy; ensure adequate hydration during therapy; ensure that patient completes full 19 days of therapy.
2.5 to 10 mg I.M., S.C., or P.O.; repeat in 12 to 48 hours if needed	Reversal takes time; protect patient from injury or invasive procedures; monitor coagulation studies; have plasma or whole blood on standby if response isn't as anticipated.

Appendix B
Antidotes for vesicant extravasation

If a vesicant extravasates, use this table to determine which antidote—and how much of it—to give your patient. In most cases, you'll infuse the antidote through the patient's existing I.V. line. Sometimes you'll use a 1-ml tuberculin syringe to give repeated subcutaneous (S.C.) injections in a circle around the infiltrated area. Use a new needle for each injection.

ANTIDOTE	PREPARATION AND DOSE	VESICANT
phentolamine	Dilute 5 to 10 mg with 10 ml of sterile saline solution for injection. Give 5 to 10 mg.	✦ dopamine ✦ nafcillin ✦ norepinephrine ✦ potassium solution ✦ teniposide ✦ total parenteral nutrition solution ✦ vinblastine ✦ vincristine ✦ vindesine
sodium thiosulfate 10%	Dilute 4 ml with 6 ml of sterile water for injection. Give 10 ml.	✦ dobutamine ✦ dopamine ✦ epinephrine ✦ metaraminol bitartrate ✦ norepinephrine ✦ cisplatin ✦ mechlorethamine

ANTIDOTE	PREPARATION AND DOSE	VESICANT
hydrocortisone sodium succinate 100 mg/ml	Give 50 to 200 mg for 25 to 50 mg of extravasate. Usually this is followed by topical hydrocortisone cream 1%.	✦ daunorubicin ✦ doxorubicin ✦ vincristine
dimethyl sulfoxide, topical	Apply to twice the size of the infiltrated area every 6 hours and let air-dry.	✦ daunorubicin ✦ doxorubicin ✦ idarubicin ✦ mitomycin

Appendix C
Dialyzable drugs

The amount of a drug removed by dialysis differs among patients and depends on several factors, including the patient's condition, the drug's properties, length of dialysis and dialysate used, rate of blood flow or dwell time, and purpose of dialysis. This chart indicates the effect of hemodialysis on selected drugs.

DRUG	LEVEL REDUCED BY HEMODIALYSIS	DRUG	LEVEL REDUCED BY HEMODIALYSIS
acetaminophen	Yes (may not influence toxicity)	aspirin	Yes
		atenolol	Yes
acyclovir	Yes	azathioprine	Yes
allopurinol	Yes	aztreonam	Yes
alprazolam	No	captopril	Yes
amikacin	Yes	carbamazepine	No
amiodarone	No	carbenicillin	Yes
amitriptyline	No	carmustine	No
amoxicillin	Yes	cefaclor	Yes
amoxicillin/ clavulanate potassium	Yes	cefadroxil	Yes
		cefamandole	Yes
amphotericin B	No	cefazolin	Yes
ampicillin	Yes	cefepime	Yes
ampicillin/ clavulanate potassium	Yes	cefonicid	Yes (by 20%)
		cefoperazone	Yes

DRUG	LEVEL REDUCED BY HEMODIALYSIS	DRUG	LEVEL REDUCED BY HEMODIALYSIS
cefotaxime	Yes	cisplatin	No
cefotetan	Yes (by 20%)	clindamycin	No
cefoxitin	Yes	clofibrate	No
ceftazidime	Yes	clonazepam	No
ceftizoxime	Yes	clonidine	No
ceftriaxone	No	clorazepate	No
cefuroxime	Yes	cloxacillin	No
cephalexin	Yes	codeine	No
cephalothin	Yes	colchicine	No
cephradine	Yes	cortisone	No
chloral hydrate	Yes	co-trimoxazole	Yes
chlorambucil	No	cyclophosphamide	Yes
chloramphenicol	Yes (very small amount)	diazepam	No
		diazoxide	No
chlordiazepoxide	No	diclofenac	No
chloroquine	No	dicloxacillin	No
chlorpheniramine	No	digoxin	No
chlorpromazine	No	diltiazem	No
chlorthalidone	No	diphenhydramine	No
cimetidine	Yes	dipyridamole	No
ciprofloxacin	Yes (by 20%)	disopyramide	Yes

DRUG	LEVEL REDUCED BY HEMODIALYSIS	DRUG	LEVEL REDUCED BY HEMODIALYSIS
doxazosin	No	gabapentin	Yes
doxepin	No	ganciclovir	Yes
doxorubicin	No	gemfibrozil	No
doxycycline	No	gentamicin	Yes
enalapril	Yes	glipizide	No
erythromycin	Yes (by 20%)	glutethimide	Yes
ethacrynic acid	No	glyburide	No
ethambutol	Yes (by 20%)	guanfacine	No
ethchlorvynol	Yes	haloperidol	No
ethosuximide	Yes	heparin	No
famotidine	No	hydralazine	No
fenoprofen	No	hydrochlorothiazide	No
flecainide	No	hydroxyzine	No
fluconazole	Yes	ibuprofen	No
flucytosine	Yes	imipenem/cilastatin	Yes
fluorouracil	Yes	imipramine	No
fluoxetine	No	indapamide	No
flurazepam	No	indomethacin	No
fosinopril	No	insulin	No
furosemide	No	irbesartan	No
		iron dextran	No

DRUG	LEVEL REDUCED BY HEMODIALYSIS	DRUG	LEVEL REDUCED BY HEMODIALYSIS
isoniazid	Yes	methotrexate	Yes
isosorbide	No	methyldopa	Yes
isradipine	No	methylprednisolone	No
kanamycin	Yes	metoclopramide	No
ketoconazole	No	metolazone	No
ketoprofen	Yes	metoprolol	No
labetalol	No	metronidazole	Yes
levofloxacin	No	mexiletine	Yes
lidocaine	No	mezlocillin	Yes
lithium	Yes	miconazole	No
lomefloxacin	No	midazolam	No
lomustine	No	minocycline	No
loracarbet	Yes	minoxidil	Yes
loratadine	No	misoprostol	No
lorazepam	No	morphine	No
mechlorethamine	No	nabumetone	No
mefenamic acid	No	nadolol	Yes
meperidine	No	nafcillin	No
mercaptopurine	Yes	naproxen	No
methadone	No	nelfinavir	Yes
methicillin	No	netilmicin	Yes

DRUG	LEVEL REDUCED BY HEMODIALYSIS	DRUG	LEVEL REDUCED BY HEMODIALYSIS
nifedipine	No	piroxicam	No
nimodipine	No	prazosin	No
nitrofurantoin	Yes	prednisone	No
nitroglycerin	No	primidone	Yes
nitroprusside	Yes	procainamide	Yes
nizatidine	No	promethazine	No
norfloxacin	No	propoxyphene	No
nortriptyline	No	propranolol	No
ofloxacin	Yes	protriptyline	No
olanzapine	No	quinidine	Yes
omeprazole	No	ranitidine	Yes
oxacillin	No	rifampin	No
oxazepam	No	rofecoxib	No
paroxetine	No	sertraline	No
penicillin G	Yes	sotalol	Yes
pentamidine	No	stavudine	Yes
pentazocine	Yes	streptomycin	Yes
phenobarbital	Yes	sucralfate	No
phenylbutazone	No	sulbactam	Yes
phenytoin	No	sulfamethoxazole	Yes
piperacillin	Yes	sulindac	No

DRUG	LEVEL REDUCED BY HEMODIALYSIS
temazepam	No
theophylline	Yes
ticarcillin	Yes
timolol	No
tobramycin	Yes
tocainide	Yes
tolbutamide	No
topiramate	Yes
trazodone	No
triazolam	No
trimethoprim	Yes
valacyclovir	Yes
valproic acid	No
valsartan	No
vancomycin	No
verapamil	No
warfarin	No

Appendix D
Adverse reactions misinterpreted as age-related changes

Some adverse reactions result from aging, drug therapy, or both. This chart lists drug classes and indicates their associated adverse reactions.

DRUG CLASSIFICATION
Alpha$_1$-adrenergic blockers
Angiotensin-converting enzyme inhibitors
Antianginals
Antiarrhythmics
Anticholinergics
Anticonvulsants
Antidepressants, tricyclic
Antidiabetics, oral
Antihistamines
Antilipemics
Antiparkinsonians
Antipsychotics
Barbiturates
Benzodiazepines
Beta blockers
Calcium channel blockers
Corticosteroids
Diuretics
Nonsteroidal anti-inflammatory drugs
Opioids
Skeletal muscle relaxants
Thyroid hormones

ADVERSE REACTION

	Agitation	Anxiety	Arrhythmias	Ataxia	Changes in appetite	Confusion	Constipation	Depression	Difficulty breathing	Disorientation	Dizziness	Drowsiness	Edema	Fatigue	Hypotension	Insomnia	Memory loss	Muscle weakness	Restlessness	Sexual dysfunction	Tremors	Urinary dysfunction	Vision changes
		◆					◆	◆			◆	◆	◆	◆	◆	◆				◆		◆	◆
					◆	◆	◆				◆			◆	◆	◆				◆			◆
	◆	◆	◆			◆					◆		◆	◆	◆	◆			◆	◆		◆	◆
				◆			◆		◆		◆		◆	◆									
	◆	◆	◆			◆	◆	◆		◆	◆	◆		◆	◆		◆	◆	◆			◆	◆
	◆		◆	◆	◆	◆	◆	◆	◆		◆	◆	◆	◆	◆	◆					◆	◆	◆
	◆	◆	◆	◆	◆	◆	◆		◆	◆	◆	◆		◆	◆	◆			◆	◆	◆	◆	◆
											◆			◆									
					◆	◆	◆			◆	◆	◆		◆							◆	◆	◆
							◆				◆			◆		◆		◆		◆		◆	◆
	◆	◆		◆	◆	◆	◆	◆		◆	◆	◆		◆	◆	◆		◆			◆	◆	◆
	◆	◆	◆	◆	◆	◆	◆	◆			◆	◆		◆	◆	◆			◆	◆	◆	◆	◆
	◆	◆	◆			◆			◆	◆		◆		◆	◆				◆				
	◆			◆		◆	◆	◆	◆	◆	◆	◆		◆		◆	◆	◆			◆	◆	◆
		◆	◆					◆	◆		◆			◆	◆		◆			◆	◆	◆	◆
		◆	◆			◆		◆			◆		◆	◆	◆	◆				◆		◆	◆
	◆				◆		◆						◆	◆		◆		◆					◆
						◆					◆			◆	◆			◆			◆		
		◆				◆	◆	◆			◆	◆		◆		◆		◆					◆
	◆	◆				◆	◆	◆	◆	◆	◆	◆		◆	◆	◆	◆		◆	◆		◆	◆
	◆	◆		◆		◆		◆			◆	◆		◆	◆	◆					◆		
			◆		◆									◆							◆		

Index